Melancholia

Melancholia is a commonly experienced feeling, and one with a long and fascinating medical history which can be charted back to antiquity. Avoiding the simplistic binary opposition of constructivism and hard realism, this book argues that melancholia was a culture-bound syndrome which thrived in the West because of the structure of Western medicine since the Ancient Greeks, and because of the West's fascination with self-consciousness. While melancholia cannot be equated with modern depression, Matthew Bell argues that concepts from recent depression research can shed light on melancholia. Within a broad historical panorama, Bell focuses on ancient medical writing, especially the little-known but pivotal Rufus of Ephesus, and on the medicine and culture of early modern Europe. Separate chapters are dedicated to issues of gender and cultural difference, and the final chapter offers a survey of melancholia in the arts, explaining the prominence of melancholia – especially in literature.

Matthew Bell is Professor of German and Comparative Literature at King's College London. His main areas of research are eighteenth-century literature and thought and the history of the human sciences, and he is the author of *The German Tradition of Psychology in Literature and Thought, 1700–1840* (Cambridge University Press, 2005).

Melancholia:
The Western Malady

Matthew Bell

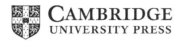
CAMBRIDGE
UNIVERSITY PRESS

CAMBRIDGE
UNIVERSITY PRESS

University Printing House, Cambridge CB2 8BS, United Kingdom

Cambridge University Press is part of the University of Cambridge.

It furthers the University's mission by disseminating knowledge in the pursuit of
education, learning and research at the highest international levels of excellence.

www.cambridge.org
Information on this title: www.cambridge.org/9781107069961

First published 2014

Printed in the United Kingdom by Clays, St Ives plc

A catalogue record for this publication is available from the British Library

ISBN 978-1-107-06996-1 Hardback

To my mother and father, whose endless generosity and kindness have made everything possible, this small token of my love and thanks.

Contents

Preface

This book developed over several years of teaching and research on melancholia in eighteenth-century Europe, during which I also tried to extend and deepen my knowledge of the long history of melancholia. Most histories tell broadly the same story. Melancholia emerged out of the highly rationalistic and systematic Ancient Greek theory of the four humours. As such, melancholia was not only a disease; it was also a temperament. Hence it made perfect sense when around 300 BC a writer of the Aristotelian school, formerly thought to be Aristotle himself, proposed that melancholia is found in all men of genius: poets, philosophers, statesmen. This theory of melancholy genius was rediscovered in the Renaissance and became the source of a major European cultural tradition, feeding into works such as Dürer's etching *Melencolia I* (1514), Shakespeare's *Hamlet* (*c.* 1601), and Goethe's novel *The Sorrows of Young Werther* (1774). In the early modern period melancholia developed a vast range of cultural expressions, at the heart of which was the conflict between our aspirations to infinity and the limitations of our actual existence. But with the advent of professional psychiatry in the nineteenth century and the eclipse of the Graeco-Roman medical tradition, this culturally rich, pre-scientific melancholia gave way to the more prosaic, but scientifically verifiable, disease of depression.

At any rate this is how melancholia has been understood since the publication of *Saturn and Melancholy*, the great reconstruction of the sources of Dürer's iconography. First conceived by Erwin Panofsky and Fritz Saxl in the early 1920s at the Warburg Library in Hamburg, and published in 1964 with substantial input from Raymond Klibansky, the book has acquired (appropriately) iconic status in the historiography of European culture and still exerts a powerful influence on studies of melancholia. Indeed, the recent growth of scholarly interest in melancholia is in large part thanks to *Saturn and Melancholy*. However, in some important respects its influence has created a misleading picture of melancholia's history. The Warburg trio saw that elements in *Melencolia I* derived from the pseudo-Aristotelian tradition of melancholy genius. However, that tradition was only ever a minor tributary of the much broader melancholy discourse, and within that broader discourse the single most important element was the tradition of medical writing on melancholia, of which the pseudo-Aristotelian text was decidedly not a part. Some recent studies have mistakenly treated *Saturn and Melancholy* as if, instead of tracing the sources of Dürer's etching, it gave a representative account of the melancholy tradition *in toto*. The result has been that the importance of genial melancholia is often overstated. Second, working with the classical scholarship available to them, Klibansky, Panofsky, and Saxl presented a rather undifferentiated picture of melancholia in antiquity. They assumed that the fully worked out tetradic humoral scheme, if not explicitly mentioned in the earliest Hippocratic texts, was at least present by implication at the birth of melancholia, so that melancholia could be seen as the offspring of this peculiarly rationalistic Ancient Greek style of thinking about human nature.[1] Subsequent work by historians of Graeco-Roman medicine has shown that this was not the case. The model of melancholia presented in the earliest Hippocratic writings was more differentiated and more empirically grounded than *Saturn and Melancholy* suggested. It will become apparent in the Introduction why I think these two issues are significant.

Saturn and Melancholy brought to light, for the first time, the full historical span of the melancholy tradition, from its beginnings in fifth-century BC Greece to its waning in the nineteenth century. This historical span presents a challenge to scholarship. Among recent studies of the history of melancholia only one has a breadth comparable to *Saturn and Melancholy*: Stanley Jackson's *Melancholia and Depression: From Hippocratic Times to Modern Times*. Jackson gives accurate and thorough accounts of the medical theories of melancholia. His book is rich in the kind of material, by turns baffling, beguiling, bizarre, and bathetic, that melancholia offers in abundance. What Jackson does not do in any systematic way is ask what melancholia actually was, and he has little to say about issues that concern recent scholarship, in particular gender and the social dimensions of melancholia. On a smaller scale, Jennifer Radden has written a series of penetrating philosophical essays on melancholia that have addressed the 'what is melancholia?' question directly. There is also a wealth of specialist literature, where the kind of historical overview provided by Jackson and the philosophical perspective of Radden's work are understandably absent, and where the impact of *Saturn and Melancholy* has often led to a skewed emphasis. Many scholars writing on modern melancholia have little knowledge of the Graeco-Roman or Arabic sources, so that some important

---

[1] See Raymond Klibansky, Erwin Panofsky, and Fritz Saxl, *Saturn and Melancholy: Studies in the History of Natural Philosophy, Religion, and Art* (New York: Basic Books, 1964), 4–13.

figures have been neglected, notably Rufus of Ephesus. Rufus was arguably the second most important figure in the Graeco-Roman discourse on melancholia, after Hippocrates. He figures prominently in Chapter 2 of this book. Having pointed out gaps in other scholars' knowledge, I am duty bound to admit a significant gap in my own. I have no Arabic, so that my discussion of Arabic sources in the following pages is second-hand or derives from translations (e.g. Karl Garbers's German edition of the *Treatise on Melancholia* by the medieval physician Isḥāq ibn ʿImrān).

My aim in this book has been to propose a new way of understanding the great tradition of melancholia in the West. But since the book grew out of a sense that a gap needed to be filled – the gap left by the rather traditional scholarship of Jackson, the philosophically informed essays of Radden, and the specialist literature – the shape of that gap has to some extent determined the shape of the book. There would have been no sense in duplicating Jackson's work by writing a narrative history of melancholia. So while this is a decidedly historical book, I decided not to organize it as a linear narrative, though parts of the early chapters are organized chronologically. Instead its organizing principle is a series of methodological questions about the nature of melancholia, which are missing from Jackson's work. Because the focus is on these methodological questions rather than on narrative history, some repetition of material has been inevitable.

In writing the book I have drawn heavily on much original work by other scholars. I make no apology for the fact that most of the originality in the book is not mine. But there is one overarching argument that I think is original. Put briefly, I want to move away from the sort of socially and economically grounded histories that interpret melancholia as an anxious reflex response to change – for instance, to the transition from a feudal and corporatist world to a capitalist and individualist one. These theories seem to me too local both chronologically and geographically to explain something as big as the Western tradition of melancholia. The passivity that these histories impute to melancholics also worries me, as I explain in Chapter 4. Instead, my interpretation draws its causal factors from the realm of ideas. As a principle of methodology, I try, where possible, to explain ideas in terms of other ideas. One distinctive feature of Western culture is the high status that it has accorded to self-consciousness. Melancholia, or at least the psychological symptoms of melancholia as reported from Hippocrates right down through Western history, depends upon the West's peculiarly introspective culture. The psychological symptoms of melancholia are, to put it crudely, a disorder of malignant self-consciousness.

Given the relatively small size of this book and the fact that it is not organized as a historical narrative, the reader should not expect anything approaching exhaustive coverage of the medical theories, let alone a full account of the broader cultural expressions of melancholia. The medical and non-medical examples I give are intended to be indicative. I try to give examples from a fairly wide range within the full chronological span of melancholia, from Hippocrates to circa 1800. As for the chronological parameters, the start date selects itself: melancholia is first attested in the earliest surviving Greek medical writings from the fifth century BC. I chose the approximate end date of 1800 for three reasons. The period around the French Revolution, or what cultural historians loosely call the Romantic period, was the deepest single rupture in European cultural history since antiquity. Much remained the same, but many of the old certainties crumbled. For instance, the tradition of Graeco-Roman medicine left only residual traces after 1800. Doctors still used a Latinized Greek nomenclature, and some of the organizing principles of medicine, both nosological and institutional, still harked back to antiquity. But the remarkably tenacious idea that physicians needed to be in continuous dialogue with the greats of Graeco-Roman medicine, Hippocrates and Galen, was finally abandoned. The period around 1800 also saw the beginnings of modern professional psychiatry. New ways of thinking about mental illness – asthenia, for example – began to replace melancholia. For strategic reasons I sometimes move beyond my end date of 1800. No study of the long history of melancholia can avoid talking about modern psychiatry's concept of depression, which is not to say that Hippocratic melancholia and contemporary depression are the same thing.

The book's geographical parameters have precisely the Western bias that its title should lead the reader to expect. The reasons for this bias are explained in Chapter 4. Within the West, I focus on the Graeco-Roman world, France, Italy, Germany, Britain, and North America. Most of the texts I examine in more detail are in Ancient Greek, English, and German, because that is where my expertise lies.

I have tried to be precise and consistent in my use of historical terminology. When talking about the medicine of classical antiquity, I use the term *Graeco-Roman*: by this I mean anything produced in the Greek and Latin linguistic area up to end of the Roman Empire in the West or up to the Byzantine Middle Ages (*c.* 1100) in the East. The term *early modern* usefully refers to the West from the end of the Middle Ages (*c.* 1400) up to around 1800. *Modern* can mean one of two things: either it refers to anything after around 1800 (so distinguishing the *modern* period from the *early modern* period), or it refers to anything since around 1400 (in which case *modern* includes *early modern* and is distinguished from antiquity and the Middle Ages). It should be clear from the context which of these two meanings applies in any given instance.

As for psychological and psychiatric terms, I initially set out to avoid using technical terminology, but became addicted to its convenience as a form of shorthand. To continue the addiction metaphor, what tends to happen is that you start with simple and innocuous words like *symptom* and then move on to harder stuff, and before you know it the habit is impossible to kick. So the reader will meet terms like *nosology* (the study of the classification of diseases), *aetiology* (the causation of disease), *pathophysiology* (the changes in bodily tissue due to disease), *pathogenesis* (the origin and development of the disease), and *epidemiology* (the study of the prevalence of diseases in human populations). Most of this terminology is concentrated in the Introduction, after which the rest of the book is written in (my version of) English, albeit with one significant exception. I have consistently preferred the Latin form *melancholia* to the Englished form *melancholy*. Some of the reasons for this are discussed in Chapter 1, but I will briefly list them here too. In the first place *melancholia* reminds us of the European character of the disease. There is a large literature focusing on English (or British) 'melancholy' of the early modern period, and this literature often gives the impression that British 'melancholy' was somehow distinctive. I am not persuaded by the arguments for the exceptionalism of British 'melancholy'. I discuss the issues surrounding national forms of melancholia in Chapter 4. It seems to me that not much is lost and quite a lot is gained by using the form *melancholia*. *Melancholia* is what linguists call a loanword, transliterated into Latin from the Ancient Greek μελαγχολία. So *melancholia* helpfully reminds us of the disease's Greek origins. It also reminds us that this is in the first place a medical matter, and only secondarily a broader cultural phenomenon. So another reason to use *melancholia* is to try to reassert the gap that originally existed between medical and non-medical discourses and that the word *melancholy* tends to obscure. Finally, a little bit of defamiliarization is a good thing. In line with my avoidance of *melancholy*, I would have liked to use the adjective *melancholic* throughout instead of *melancholy*, but that was a linguistic bridge too far. *Melancholic* is used (more or less consistently) as an adjectival noun to refer to a person suffering from *melancholia*.

In his *Anatomy of Melancholy*, first published in 1621 and then in four further editions, each more capacious than the one before, Robert Burton complained of the superabundance of books spewing from the presses every year. (As is often the case with Burton, he does precisely what he warns us against.) And he bemoaned his own fate as a recycler of other men's words, words that were his own and not his own:

[W]ee shall have a vast *Chaos* and confusion of Bookes, we are oppressed with them, our eyes ake with reading, our fingers with turning. For my part I am one of the number, *nos numerus sumus* [we are mere ciphers]: I doe not denie it, I have only this of *Macrobius* to say for my selfe, *Omne meum, nihil meum,* 'tis all mine, and none mine.[2]

There are now many more books than there were in Burton's day, and many more books on melancholia. This book is quite like all the ones that have gone before, and also a bit different.

---

[2] Robert Burton, *The Anatomy of Melancholy*, ed. Thomas C. Faulkner *et al.*, 5 vols. (Oxford University Press, 1989), vol. I, 'Democritus to the Reader', 11.

Acknowledgements

In the first place would like to thank my colleagues and students in the Departments of German and Comparative Literature at King's College London. In particular, students on my MA course 'Melancholia and hypochondria in eighteenth-century European literature' have indulged my unhealthy fascination with the subject and provided the best self-help group one could ask for.

In 2011 King's played host to a remarkably diverse and interesting group of guests and speakers for a conference on religious melancholy. The conference was generously funded by the Wellcome Trust.

Various parts of this project have been given outings before appreciative audiences at the following institutions: California State University Long Beach; the English Goethe Society, London; the Institute of Germanic and Romance Studies, London; the Institute of Psychiatry, London; the Jawaharlal Nehru University, New Delhi; the University of North Carolina at Chapel Hill; and the universities of Cambridge, Northumbria, Oxford, Sheffield, and Stuttgart.

I would like to be able to remember all the conversations about melancholia I have had with friends and colleagues, and to acknowledge them here. Sadly my memory is deficient and the list, long though it would be, would contain too many omissions. So I will confine myself to recording special thanks to the following colleagues for their generous help and expertise: Eric Gidal, Simon Glendinning, Angus Gowland, Jeremy Schmidt, Michael Silk, and Neil Vickers. Cambridge University Press recruited six anonymous reviewers who gave extensive and thoughtful comments on the typescript. Jennifer Radden and Julius Rubin, both of whom know much more about melancholia than I do, were especially generous with their help. I have followed some of their suggestions, and the book is better for them; if I had followed all of them, it would be better still. Throughout the writing of the book, I have been encouraged and inspired by my dear friend and colleague Jane Darcy.

The team at Cambridge University Press, Hetty Marx, Rebecca Taylor, and Christina Sarigiannidou, have been faultlessly efficient, professional, and a pleasure to work with. Joseph Garver has edited with care and wisdom. I am sincerely grateful to them.

Love and thanks go to my family: Lou, Florence, Cecily, Meg, Pete, Sarah, Christine. John Weston Smith is missed terribly. I like to think he would have enjoyed the book; I know it would be wittier and more stylish if he had written it.

Note on citation, quotation, translation, and spelling

Full references to all sources are included in the footnotes to each chapter, and all sources used are listed in the bibliography, with the following exceptions. For Graeco-Roman and biblical texts, where established conventions of reference exist (e.g. Plato, *Apology*, 38a, or Leviticus 15:19–30, 20), I have used these established conventions. For these texts it would have been superfluous to provide references to specific editions, and I have not done so, nor are these texts listed in the bibliography. I have made an exception to this rule for some texts that are of particular importance to the history of melancholia, notably the Graeco-Roman medical texts. In Chapter 2, where I give an extended account of the theories of Rufus of Ephesus, I have included references to Rufus' fragments in the main body of my text.

All foreign-language texts are quoted in English. In most cases, the footnotes and bibliography provide details of easily available translations of these texts. Where no translation exists or the existing translations are adequate or easily available, the translations are my own.

The spelling of pre-modern texts has been preserved; or, to be more precise, I have used the spelling given in the editions from which I quote. Names of classical authors are given in their traditional English forms. On occasions where Greek words are transliterated, I have used $\bar{e}$ and $\bar{o}$ to stand for *eta* and *omega* respectively (i.e. a long *e* and long *o*).

Introduction

1   The persistence of melancholia

Lars von Trier's 2011 feature film *Melancholia* tells the story of two sisters, the incorrigibly chaotic, selfish, and depressed Justine, played by Kirsten Dunst, and the organized, calm, and caring Claire (Charlotte Gainsbourg).[1] Or that is how they behave in the first half of the film, titled 'Justine'. In the second half, 'Claire', they seem to swap characters, and it is Claire who is erratic, anxious, and self-centred. A mysterious planet Melancholia is menacingly approaching the Earth. Governments and scientists have assured the public that Melancholia will fly past harmlessly, but Justine believes what she reads in the wilder reaches of the internet: that the planets will collide and Earth will be destroyed. Sure enough Melancholia passes close by and then whips back in a 'slingshot' orbit on a collision course with Earth. In the face of catastrophe the previously calm and rational Claire becomes agitated, erratic, and self-obsessed. The melancholic Justine, on the other hand, attains a state of calm and is able to comfort Claire's young son Leo at the end of all things. Von Trier has suggested that the film developed out of his own experience of depression, and in particular the insight that those who, like Justine, suffer from depression are able to respond calmly to crises, perhaps because their pessimism has prepared them for the worst.[2] But von Trier chose the title *Melancholia*, not *Depression*. The word *depression* never occurs in the film, though the diagnosis of depression would surely be part of the ordinary lexicon of the film's educated, wealthy characters – educated, but seemingly in denial. Perhaps the word *depression* is absent because the characters are set on denying its existence, in the same way as most of them will deny that Melancholia is on a collision course with Earth. The planet Melancholia thus has a metaphorical function in von Trier's film, both standing for depression and standing in an oddly oblique relation to it.

---

[1] *Melancholia*, film dir. by Lars von Trier (Zentropa, 2011).
[2] www.dfi.dk/Service/English/News-and-publications/FILM-Magazine/Artikler-fra-tidsskriftet-FILM/72/The-Only-Redeeming-Factor-is-the-World-Ending.aspx.

The idea of melancholia is around 2,500 years old at least. Its earliest surviving appearance is in the writings of Hippocrates of Cos (*c.* 460–*c.* 370 BC) and his school. After Hippocrates melancholia enjoyed a long and unchallenged reign within the terminology, nosology, and practice of mental medicine, until it was eclipsed by depression in the early twentieth century. Von Trier's *Melancholia* is one of a number of recent works that return to the ancient idea of melancholia in order to find new ways to talk about what we now call depression. Indeed, one of the functions of melancholia in von Trier's film is to disturb our common-sense, folk-psychological understanding of depression, to show us that there is more to depression than just low mood and self-loathing, and that melancholia can have positive attributes. In current psychiatry too, there is evidence of unease with depression and a desire to return to melancholia, albeit for quite different reasons. In their 2006 book *Melancholia: The Diagnosis, Pathophysiology, and Treatment of Depressive Illness*, the American neuro-psychiatrists Michael Alan Taylor and Max Fink propose that melancholia be reinstated as a medical diagnosis.[3] In a 2007 article Edward Shorter, a leading historian of psychiatry, argues that the diagnosis of major depressive disorder should be replaced by two separate forms of depressive disorder, 'melancholic mood disorder' and 'non-melancholic mood disorder', a distinction introduced by the Australian psychopathologist Gordon Parker.[4] In June 2010 a group of psychiatrists, including Parker, Taylor, and Fink, published an editorial in the *American Journal of Psychiatry* arguing that the American Psychiatric Association's taxonomy of mental disorders should recognize melancholia as a separate major disorder, alongside and distinct from depression.[5]

How do we explain this continuing interest, both cultural and scientific, in an idea that seemed to have passed into obsolescence a hundred years ago? The Hippocratic writings give several accounts of the illness. It was a grave mental and physical affliction, with profound effects on emotion, cognition, and physical health. For instance, in a case recorded in the Hippocratic *Epidemics*, a woman of Thasos was said to be suffering from 'coma ... aversion to food, despondency, sleeplessness, irritability,

---

[3] Michael Alan Taylor and Max Fink, *Melancholia: The Diagnosis, Pathophysiology and Treatment of Depressive Illness* (Cambridge University Press, 2006).

[4] Edward Shorter, 'The Doctrine of the Two Depressions in Historical Perspective', *Acta Psychiatrica Scandinavica* 115, suppl. 433 (2007), 5–13. See also Shorter, *Before Prozac: The Troubled History of Mood Disorders in Psychiatry* (Oxford University Press, 2009), 165, and Gordon Parker, 'Editorial: Commentary on Diagnosing Major Depressive Disorder', *Journal of Nervous and Mental Disease* 194 (2006), 155–7.

[5] Gordon Parker *et al.*, 'Issues for DSM-5: Whither Melancholia? The Case for Its Classification as a Distinct Mood Disorder', *American Journal of Psychiatry* 167 (2010), 745–7.

restlessness [*dysphoriai*], the mind being affected by melancholia'.[6] Another case mentions strange and terrifying dreams.[7] The symptoms of Hippocratic melancholia bear comparison with the diagnosis of major depressive disorder in the latest edition of the American Psychiatric Association's *Diagnostic and Statistical Manual of Mental Disorders* (DSM-5, 2013). DSM-5 gives the following symptoms for major depressive disorder: depressed mood; diminished interest in otherwise pleasurable activities; significant weight loss or gain; insomnia or hypersomnia; psychomotor agitation or retardation; fatigue or loss of energy; feelings of worthlessness or guilt; diminished ability to think or concentrate; recurrent thoughts of death.[8] If we allow for their different modes of expression and for different cultural norms, Hippocrates and DSM-5 show several similarities: both refer to low mood, disturbances of sleep and diet, agitation, and lethargy. This has led Stanley Jackson to conclude that there is a 'remarkable continuity' in the psychological symptoms of ancient melancholia and modern depression.[9] To be sure, the contrary case can also be made; even from this purely descriptive perspective, in other words without considering the ontology of the disease, we might conclude that the differences outweigh the similarities.[10] Jackson acknowledges that the disorders labelled melancholia and depression have changed in significant ways over time. For instance, the range of conditions covered by melancholia up to the early modern period was far greater than that covered by modern depression.[11] And he acknowledges that in the modern period numerous very different physiological models have been used to explain the phenomena – 'a parade of theories', as he puts it.[12] But having acknowledged these changes, he sticks to his thesis of a 'remarkable continuity'.

2   Psychiatric realism and constructivism

The most obvious, and I think the most compelling, way of accounting for Jackson's continuity would be a form of psychiatric realism. We

---

[6] *Epidemics*, iii, 17, 2, in *Hippocrates I*, trans. W. H. S. Jones, Loeb Classical Library (London: Heinemann, 1948), 263.

[7] Hippocrates, *De morbis*, cited by Helmut Flashar, *Melancholie und Melancholiker in den medizinischen Theorien der Antike* (Berlin: de Gruyter, 1966), 51.

[8] American Psychiatric Association, *Diagnostic and Statistical Manual of Mental Disorders*, 5th edn (DSM-5) (Arlington, VA: APA, 2013), 160–1.

[9] Stanley Jackson, *Melancholia and Depression: From Hippocratic Times to Modern Times* (New Haven, CT: Yale University Press, 1986), *passim*.

[10] Jennifer Radden, 'Is This Dame Melancholy? Equating Today's Depression and Past Melancholia', *Philosophy, Psychiatry, &Psychology* 10 (2003), 37–52.

[11] Jackson, *Melancholia*, 399.   [12] *Ibid.*, 386–90.

would want to say that, having allowed for cultural differences in their forms of expression, Hippocratic melancholia and DSM-5-style depression represent the observable phenomena of one and the same disorder. Melancholia and depression have features in common because they both represent the structure of a single reality. Clearly things are not that simple. During their long history melancholia and depression have not always represented the same facets of that reality or represented it with equal clarity. We might also wonder what level of reality they represent. Are melancholia and depression labels for a set of commonly co-occurring symptoms (low mood, sleep disturbance, etc.)? In other words, is it a reality at the level of symptomatic phenomena? Or do they describe a deeper level of reality, like physiological diseases? Are they the psychiatric equivalent of diseases like influenza, each with its own specific causes, pathogenesis, physiological location, and course? The latter form of psychiatric realism might invoke an even stronger argument to the effect that melancholia and depression are 'natural kinds'. That is to say, individual instances of melancholia and depression are members of a stable and discrete set, all of whose members share the same significant properties. Questions of this kind – what exactly do we mean by *psychiatric realism*? – need not concern us just yet. (They are discussed at some length in sections 4 to 7 of this Introduction.) Whatever kind of realism they espouse, realists will argue that the theories of melancholia and depression have persisted because in some fashion and at some level they represent the structure of reality. This is indeed the view that Jackson himself takes. In spite of the theoretical variety he finds in the history of melancholia and depression, he maintains that melancholia and depression represent facts about human nature. The concluding words of his book are, 'with such distress, we are at the very heart of being human'.[13]

Psychiatric realism has been challenged by various forms of psychiatric constructivism (or constructionism). These have ranged from the radical antipsychiatry movement led by Thomas Szasz and historical constructivists such as Michel Foucault, to those who, like Ian Hacking and Mikkel Borch-Jacobsen, have positioned themselves somewhere between realism and constructivism.[14] We will return to the moderate styles of constructivism in due course. The more radical forms of constructivism centre on two

[13] *Ibid.*, 404.
[14] Szasz's publications in this field are too numerous to list here. Key works by other writers include Michel Foucault, *History of Madness* (London: Routledge, 2006); Mikkel Borch-Jacobsen, *Making Minds and Madness: From Hysteria to Depression* (Cambridge University Press, 2009); Ian Hacking, *Rewriting the Soul: Multiple Personality and the Sciences of Memory* (Princeton University Press, 1995), and *Mad Travellers: Reflections on the Reality of Transient Mental Illness* (Charlottesville, VA: University Press of Virginia, 1998).

arguments. The first concerns the nature of truth claims in psychiatry. Foucault and Szasz have both maintained that psychiatry is not a true science. They do not deny the truth claims of other sciences (e.g. chemistry and biology), but because psychiatry is uniquely implicated in complex questions of human behaviour, it cannot be properly scientific.

Taking his lead from Heidegger, Foucault consistently argued that there is no such thing as an essence of human nature. What we call 'human nature' is formed by whatever self-interpretations and social practices happen to be current in a given period. Therefore, a *science* of human nature cannot exist; all we can have is a description of the structure of historical human self-interpretations. Szasz shares the view that psychiatric science is an impossibility. This is because the phenomena that mental disorders purport to explain are in fact socio-behavioural, and not medical problems. As Szasz writes of psychiatric diagnoses such as schizophrenia, 'each of these terms refers to behaviour, not disease; to disapproved conduct, not histopathological change'.[15] Szasz acknowledges that people suffer from real distress, but he would prefer that we talked about 'problems in living' rather than mental disorders.

The constructivism of Foucault and Szasz can be contrasted with the 'strong programme' in the sociology of science initiated by David Bloor. According to the strong programme, science is to be understood as a product of the social structure of scientific communities.[16] Foucault and Szasz, by contrast, have focused on wider political questions rather than the details of the sociology of scientific institutions. Broadly speaking, both are (or became) libertarians: they argue that the weakness and indeed the *danger* of psychiatry lie in its inability to liberate itself from the state. During the early modern period, while true sciences, like physics, were growing to full maturity and attaining a measure of autonomy, psychiatry continued under the tutelage of the state. Consequently, the state was able to exploit psychiatry as a means of social control. In his *Folie et déraison* (1961; translated as *History of Madness*, 2006) Foucault argued that in the early modern period the mad, along with the sick, idle, and unemployed, were lumped together under the category of 'unreason' and confined in asylums. Psychiatry was a means of policing undesirable elements in society. It was not really *psychiatry* in any proper sense at all, since it classed many behaviours as unreason that were patently not mental disorders. Psychiatry was therefore not concerned with treating the mentally ill, but with maintaining the social and political status quo.

---

[15] Thomas Szasz, *Schizophrenia: The Sacred Symbol of Psychiatry* (Syracuse, NY: Syracuse University Press, 1988), 10.

[16] David Bloor, *Knowledge and Social Imagery* (London: Routledge & Kegan Paul, 1976), 7.

In a similar vein, Szasz has argued that psychiatry has become a tool of the modern 'therapeutic state'.[17] The state has used psychiatry to define, psychologize, and correct behaviours of which it disapproves – 'problems in living' such as suicide, unhappiness, anxiety, and shyness. For both Foucault and Szasz, then, behind psychiatry's apparently scientific diagnoses lies a complex covert web of socio-political motivations.

At this point it is helpful to distinguish between two meanings of social construction: the social construction of beliefs, and the social construction of facts.[18] By socially constructed beliefs I mean beliefs that for whatever reason cannot be tested against reality and can therefore only be explained in terms of the interests of the people who hold them. According to Foucault and Szasz, mental disorders are socially constructed beliefs. People may have had compelling social or political reasons for thinking in terms of, say, melancholia – Foucault certainly thinks this is the case – but these reasons were not rational, and the resultant beliefs were not empirically verifiable. By socially constructed facts I mean real entities that are the product of human activity. They include such things as money, the English language, and the law. No one denies that such socially constructed facts are facts. What we mean by calling them socially constructed is that they are the way they are because humans have made them so. And they might conceivably have been made quite differently; indeed, they evidently have been made differently at different times and in different places. The dispute between psychiatric realists (Jackson) and psychiatric constructivists (Foucault and Szasz) is not a dispute over whether mental disorders are socially constructed facts. Realists and constructivists should be able to agree that the phenomena covered by the psychiatric label *depression* are socially constructed facts. Cases of depression may have been caused by social factors, and the symptoms may be expressed through socially dysfunctional behaviour. For these reasons depression might indeed have been different in different places and times, depending on the different causal factors that were in play. The disagreement between realists and constructivists concerns whether depression and other psychiatric kinds are socially constructed beliefs, beliefs that are by their very nature untestable and unverifiable. The constructivists maintain that psychiatric kinds are untestable socially constructed beliefs. The realists believe that they can be tested and shown to be real.

---

[17] Thomas Szasz, *Law, Liberty, and Psychiatry: An Inquiry into the Social Uses of Mental Health Practices* (New York: Macmillan, 1963).

[18] Paul A. Boghossian, 'What Is Social Construction?', *Times Literary Supplement* 5108 (23 February 2001), 6–8.

3   Are psychiatric natural kinds possible?

Faced by the radical constructivist challenge, psychiatric realism needs to demonstrate the possibility of psychiatric natural kinds. Natural kinds play an important role in scientific realism. A realist view of science holds that, when all goes well, science is able to reveal the ways nature organizes itself into kinds such as chemical elements or biological species. It is by isolating natural kinds that science is able successfully to theorize and make inferences. The theories and inferences might involve law-like statements about causal properties of kinds. Natural kinds also form the basis of any scientific taxonomy, such as the periodic table of elements or the Linnaean taxonomy of biological species. In denying scientific status to psychiatry, Foucault and Szasz imply that there are no natural kinds in psychiatry. They insist on a contrast between psychiatry, which cannot have natural kinds, and other sciences, such as chemistry and biology, which can.

Constructivist challenges to psychiatric realism have generally aimed to show that on four key points psychiatric classifications are fundamentally unsatisfactory compared to the true natural kinds of chemistry, biology, etc.:

1. Psychiatric taxonomy is arbitrary, because psychiatry is undecided about which sets of facts constitute the basis for a diagnosis. Is diagnosis based on a disorder's symptoms or its causes or its course or its method of treatment? Each of these approaches is currently used in psychiatry, with no agreement about which of them is the decisive one.

2. In contrast with, say, chemical natural kinds (elements), psychiatric classifications are not distinguished from one another by clear boundaries. Chemical elements occupy a taxonomic space called the periodic table. Any given element has a determinate place within this space, by virtue of its atomic number. There can be no boundary disputes in the periodic table. Psychiatry by contrast is plagued by seemingly endless and irresolvable boundary disputes.

3. Psychiatry is historically mutable. As human behaviour has changed, so too psychiatric diagnoses have changed. But natural kinds ought to be more or less immutable.

4. Psychiatry studies human behaviour, which is a product of human actions. Psychiatric kinds, whatever they are, are human-made kinds, not naturally occurring ones, like nitrogen, say.

Sections 4 to 7 address these charges, outlining some of the responses psychiatric realists have made to constructivism. The aim is to show that in contrasting, say, chemical or biological kinds with psychiatric kinds the radical constructivists create a falsely binary picture of science and an unwarrantedly pessimistic view of the status of psychiatry. The distinction drawn by radical constructivism between psychiatry and 'real' science is much less clear than the constructivists suppose. This argument takes two forms. It aims to demonstrate that kinds in psychiatry are more robust than the constructivists imagine. And it aims to demonstrate that natural kinds in biology and chemistry, while possible, are less robust than the arguments of the constructivists imply. In combination these two arguments aim to show that the kinds found in chemistry, biology, and psychiatry exist on a continuum of difference. The differences between chemical, biological, and psychiatric kinds are differences in the degree of their stability. In psychiatry, as in chemistry and biology, kinds are able to support reliable inference and law-like statements. In each science, kinds possess this power to the extent that the systems in which they operate are stable ones. Gold behaves like gold, and not like nitrogen, always and everywhere in any system created by the big bang. Wolves behave like wolves, and not tigers, always and everywhere within any system containing the wolf genome and a suitable and stable ecological niche. The same applies, *mutatis mutandis*, for mental disorders.

Sections 8 to 10 address the second type of social construction: socially constructed facts. If mental disorders are natural kinds, does this not imply that they cannot be socially constructed facts? Must psychiatric natural kinds not be organic pathologies rooted in, say, brain chemistry and quite unaffected by social causation? I will follow those who, like Dominic Murphy, have argued to the contrary that the dichotomy between mental disorders as natural kinds and mental disorders as socially constructed facts is another false dichotomy.[19] To argue that mental disorders have an organic component is not to argue for complete biological reductionism. A mental disorder with an organic component can very well have social causes too. As Murphy puts it, 'debates about whether mental disorders are natural or social kinds are beside the point: they can be natural kinds even if part of their explanations is social'.[20] Sections 8 to 10 will sketch a model for combining organic and social understandings of mental disorders. Most of the argument in sections 4 onwards is unoriginal; it draws on recent work in the philosophy of psychiatry by Murphy, Ian Hacking, and others.[21] The original and distinctive part of the argument

---

[19] Dominic Murphy, *Psychiatry in the Scientific Image* (Cambridge, MA: MIT Press, 2006).

[20] *Ibid.*, 279–80.

[21] In particular I draw on Murphy, *Psychiatry in the Scientific Image*; Rachel Cooper, 'Why Hacking Is Wrong About Human Kinds', *British Journal of the Philosophy of Science* 55 (2004), 73–85; Peter Zachar, 'Psychiatric Disorders Are Not Natural Kinds', *Philosophy, Psychiatry, &Psychology* 7 (2000), 167–82, and 'Psychiatry, Scientific Laws, and Realism About Entities', in Kenneth S. Kendler and Josef Parnas (eds.), *Philosophical Issues in*

comes in section 10. There I propose a new way of understanding the socio-historical 'niche' in which melancholia developed in Europe.

For the purposes of the following sections, I am going to make three assumptions that will help to bring the realism debate into sharper focus. These assumptions are questionable, and I make them only for the temporary purposes of this Introduction.

1. I will assume that melancholia and depression are paradigmatic instances of mental disorders. This is questionable on two counts. As I suggested above, it might be more rational to think of melancholia and depression not as disorders but as symptoms – either symptoms of an underlying mental disorder or of several different disorders that share similar symptomatic profiles. If melancholia and depression turned out to be merely symptoms, it would not invalidate the search for natural kinds in psychiatry. It would only mean that we had been looking for natural kinds in the wrong place. Second, historians of antiquity will point out that in much of the medical writing melancholia has more in common with a physical disease than a mental disorder, and that in some of the ancient sources it has no mental symptoms at all.[22] While this is undeniably true, my argument concerns the *potential* of melancholia to be classified as a mental disorder, not whether all forms of it ought to be so classified.

2. Connected with the first assumption, I will also assume that a mental disorder is a discrete entity, like a disease in general medicine. Again this might be wrong. It might be that none of the disorder concepts in psychiatry (depression, anxiety, schizophrenia, etc.) are discrete entities, but instead are all the varied expressions of a single, very broad psychiatric malaise.

3. I will assume that Stanley Jackson is right in supposing that melancholia and depression are different representations of the same thing. So in the following sections melancholia and depression will almost always appear yoked together, or when I use one term the other can usually be taken as implied.

I should stress that these three assumptions do not hold good outside this introductory chapter. Their function is only to give clarity to the issues surrounding the realism debate. I should also stress that in using the term *depression* in these introductory pages I am referring to a composite object, not to a historically determinate understanding of depression. I am not referring specifically to the definition of major depressive episode or major

---

Psychiatry (Baltimore, MD: Johns Hopkins University Press, 2008), 39–47 (at pp. 39–42); Muhammad Ali Khalidi, 'Interactive Kinds', *British Journal for the Philosophy of Science* 61 (2010), 335–60.

[22] Jackie Pigeaud, '*Prolégomènes* à une histoire de la mélancolie', *Histoire, économie et société* 3 (1984), 501–10 (at p. 502).

depressive disorder in DSM-5, or the similar depressive episode and recurrent depressive disorder in the World Health Organization's *International Classification of Disease* (ICD-10, 1988), or the depression constructs of the rating scales most commonly used by clinicians and researchers (the Hamilton Rating Scale for Depression and the Beck Depression Inventory). I have in mind something rather broader, which encompasses these definitions – namely, the general usage of *depression* in modern psychiatric practice and research. The fact that the various constructs of depression listed above are not in complete agreement is not relevant to my argument, nor is the question of whether a composite concept such as I have just outlined here (as distinct from any particular depression construct) can be said to be meaningful. My argument concerns the *possibility* of psychiatric natural kinds, not what any actual psychiatric natural kind looks like. The same applies to my use of the term *melancholia* in this Introduction. In subsequent chapters I will be talking about historically determinate meanings of the term *melancholia*. But in this Introduction I have in mind a composite concept that includes a wide range of the term's historical meanings as well as its uses in contemporary psychiatry.

4   Taxonomy

How should the phenomena of melancholia and depression be classified? As I have already suggested, there is more than one factual resource on which we could ground a taxonomy of mental disorders, and the different factual resources can be made to generate quite different disease constructs. For instance, one might prefer a purely symptom-based taxonomy, and one might accordingly choose to remain agnostic about whether depression is a discrete disorder or merely a set of symptoms of some broader underlying disorder. In this spirit some researchers have argued that the medical model of discrete disease categories is inappropriate for psychiatry, and that instead we should think in terms of a smaller number of disorders which express themselves in diverse ways.[23] (This approach to classification is sometimes termed 'lumping', as opposed to 'splitting' into more and smaller categories.) Most attempts at psychiatric classification involve a higher degree of splitting. One approach is to define disorders in terms of stable sets of co-occurring symptoms that follow a regular course. This approach does not involve any claims about the causation and organic nature of the disease; it simply records the patterns of co-occurring symptoms and their course over

---

[23] See, for example, Richard P. Bentall, *Madness Explained: Psychosis and Human Nature* (Harmondsworth: Penguin, 2004).

time. This descriptive approach is the one favoured by DSM-III and its subsequent revisions. To quote DSM-III:

This approach can be said to be 'descriptive' in that the definitions of the disorders generally consist of descriptions of the clinical features of the disorders. The features are described at the lowest order of inference necessary to describe the characteristic features of the disorder.[24]

According to this view, psychiatrists can be agnostic about the nature of any underlying neurochemical or neurobiological processes. What matters is that a meaningful cluster of symptoms occur together and follow a distinct course. An emphasis on the course of the illness has traditionally been thought to justify this approach. Emil Kraepelin argued that '*only the overall picture of a medical case from the beginning to the end of its development* can provide justification for its being linked with other observations of the same kind'.[25] Finally, some splitters are not content with the ontological agnosticism of Kraepelin and DSM. These stronger forms of psychiatric taxonomy will want to consider the causes of disorders and their underlying neurobiology and neurochemistry.

In other words, different factual resources may yield quite different schemes of classification. The problem of multiple factual resources is not unique to psychiatry. Biological classification faces similar difficulties. The common and intuitive assumption, dating from Aristotle, was that biological species were paradigmatic instances of natural kinds. Recent developments in biology have made this assumption harder to sustain. Traditional definitions of biological species – the Linnaean definition based on morphological properties, or the idea of species as reproductively isolated populations – have proved unable to resolve a host of boundary disputes. Genetics promised a more reliable definition of the species concept, but biologists still find the more traditional methods of classification provide help where genetics is found wanting. Each of these three factual resources may be useful to the biologist and may reveal a similar though not necessarily identical classification of species. The fact that biologists use three different factual resources that do not overlap exactly does not mean we should jettison realism about species – the classifications arrived at by these various means do reflect the structure of nature. But it is a 'promiscuous realism', as John Dupré terms it, since it allows the biologist to appeal to different factual resources – genetics,

---

[24] American Psychiatric Association, *Diagnostic and Statistical Manual of Mental Disorders*, 3rd edn (DSM-III) (Washington, DC: APA, 1980), 7.

[25] Emil Kraepelin, *Psychiatry: A Textbook for Students and Physicians*, 6th edn, reprint (Canton, MA: Science History Publications, 1990), 3.

morphology, reproductive isolation – in order to define a given species concept.[26] Similar considerations might apply to the various factual resources used to define mental disorders: symptoms, causes, course, and underlying neurophysiology.

5   Boundary disputes

In the periodic table of chemical elements the kinds are bounded, exhaustive, and non-overlapping. There are no gaps between taxonomic spaces, no elements that do not fall into a single taxonomic space, and no spaces that are occupied by more than one element. Consequently, there are no boundary disputes. Psychiatry, by contrast, is riddled with boundary disputes. Often diagnosis of a psychiatric case is difficult because the case concurrently displays symptoms associated with more than one disorder. As a consequence, one psychiatrist will diagnose quite differently from another. Numerous studies have shown that reliability of diagnosis in psychiatry – the tendency of a given set of symptoms to generate the same diagnosis from more than one psychiatrist – is worryingly low and considerably lower than in general medicine.[27]

Another cause of boundary disputes in psychiatry is the problem of comorbidity. In general medicine, comorbidity is defined as the coexistence of two or more distinct diseases in a patient. They might be unrelated diseases (lung cancer and diabetes), or unrelated diseases in or near the same organ (breast cancer and respiratory infections), or distinct disorders with a shared causal factor (type-2 diabetes and hypertension, both caused by obesity). Comorbidity is a complex field in general medicine, but it is even more fraught in psychiatry because it seems to be so common.[28] Large-scale studies of mental disorders in the USA have shown that comorbidity is the rule rather than the exception. The most frequent instance of psychiatric comorbidity is the coexistence of depression and anxiety; these two disorders occur more frequently together than they do apart. In the US National Comorbidity Survey, conducted from 1990 to 1992, over 50 per cent of people in the community qualifying for a DSM-III diagnosis of depression also

[26] John Dupré, 'Natural Kinds and Biological Taxa', *Philosophical Review* 90 (1981), 66–90 (at p. 82).

[27] See especially J. E. Cooper *et al.*, *Psychiatric Diagnosis in New York and London* (Oxford University Press, 1972). For further studies, see Bentall, *Madness Explained*, 44–56.

[28] Richard J. McNally, *What Is Mental Illness?* (Cambridge, MA: Harvard University Press, 2011), 185.

qualified for a diagnosis of an anxiety disorder.[29] A study of patients attending primary care found a 75 per cent rate of comorbidity for depression and anxiety.[30] These studies suggest that, while they form separate diagnostic categories in DSM, depression and anxiety might in fact be different expressions of the same underlying disorder. (DSM-5 includes 'with anxious distress' as a features specifier of depressive disorders; this reflects the fact of this comorbidity, though it does little to resolve the larger nosological problem posed by the very extensive comorbidity of anxiety and depression.)[31]

A second form of boundary dispute concerns the threshold at which a condition becomes a disease or, as DSM-IV-TR puts it, the threshold that separates a mental disorder 'from no mental disorder at all'.[32] Arguably, the problem of blurred thresholds affects many mental disorders. The symptoms of depression affect many perfectly healthy people at lower levels or transiently after suffering loss or stress. At what threshold do these symptoms cease to be normal and become pathological? While it might seem that the threshold problem makes psychiatric diagnosis arbitrary, the same issue affects many physical disorders in general medicine. Some diseases are pathological extensions of normally occurring and harmless states. For instance, primary hypertension is diagnosed when a patient's blood pressure exceeds 140/90 mmHg. The threshold for a diagnosis of hypertension is based on statistical evidence, but the statistical evidence takes the form of a smooth gradient, not a sudden step.

Psychiatry is by no means alone in suffering from boundary disputes. Boundary disputes are simply endemic to any biological kinds. Biological species have long been cited as paradigmatic cases of natural kindhood, but they suffer from boundary disputes as much as psychiatry does. The traditional methods used to classify biological species – morphology and reproductive isolation – were bedevilled by boundary disputes. Related biological species are sometimes morphologically identical. The Scottish crossbill, a small, sparrow-like bird, was confirmed as a separate species in 2006 on the basis of its distinct calls, but it is morphologically indistinguishable from the common crossbill and parrot

[29] R. C. Kessler, C. Nelson, K. A. McGonagle, et al., 'Comorbidity of DSM-III-R Major Depressive Disorder in the General Population: Results from the US National Comorbidity Survey', British Journal of Psychiatry 168, suppl. 30 (1996), 17–30.
[30] M. Olfson, B. Fireman, M. M. Weissman, et al., 'Mental Disorders and Disability Among Patients in a Primary Care Group Practice', American Journal of Psychiatry 154 (1997), 1734–40.
[31] American Psychiatric Association, DSM-5, 184.
[32] American Psychiatric Association, Diagnostic and Statistical Manual of Mental Disorders, 4th edn; text rev. (DSM-IV-TR) (Washington, DC: APA, 2000), xxxi. See also McNally, Mental Illness, 47–54.

crossbill.[33] Reproductive isolation suffers from similar difficulties. Many morphologically and genetically distinct species are able successfully to interbreed and produce non-sterile offspring. Any birdwatcher will be able to confirm that successful interbreeding between related species is relatively common, as, for instance, in gulls and ducks

Genetics promised a more reliable definition of the biological species concept. Now a species could be defined in terms of a genome, with precise quantitative data. But far from overcoming boundary disputes, genetics threw up new and equally intractable ones. Populations of organisms contain considerable degrees of genetic variation. But how do we decide what degree of genetic variation is permissible within a single species? Whatever degree of variation we settle for, the definition of a species will be established not by categorical distinctions, but by statistical variables, just like our example of hypertension above. Hence species would not be distinct in the sense required by the strong notion of a natural kind outlined above – that is, the requirement that the divisions between natural kinds are categorical breaks and not smooth transitions. Even if most species were distinguished from one another fairly clearly, there would always be instances of populations that were not so easily distinguishable, so at some point the notion of species as natural kinds would always be liable to break down.

Even so, it might still be possible to recover a workable version of biological natural kinds. Clearly, biological species cannot be defined in terms of any essential properties that form necessary and sufficient conditions for kindhood. Instead of reducing them to essences, we can define species in terms of clusters of properties. Dupré has argued that from the perspective of genetics, biological species may be thought to occupy more or less tight clusters of individuals.[34] For instance, if we imagine biological individuals as occupying points in genetic space, the members of a species will crowd around a central point. Although there will be some diffuseness and a few rogue outliers, each cluster of related individuals will be separated from neighbouring clusters by some empty or sparsely populated space. As much as anything, it is the difference between densely and sparsely populated space that creates confidence in the possibility of biological natural kinds. In principle a similar approach could be applied to mental disorders.

---

[33] R. W. Summers, R. J. Dawson, and R. E. Phillips, 'Assortative Mating and Patterns of Inheritance Indicate That the Three Crossbill Taxa in Scotland Are Species', *Journal of Avian Biology* 38 (2007), 153–62.

[34] Dupré, 'Natural Kinds and Biological Taxa', 66–90; see also by the same author, *The Disorder of Things: Metaphysical Foundations of the Disunity of Science* (Cambridge, MA: Harvard University Press, 1993), 15–84.

6   **Mutability**

One of the constructivists' main objections to psychiatric realism is that psychiatric categories lack the temporal invariability of categories in the natural sciences. Chemical natural kinds are invariable and immutable: the kind nitrogen is the same no matter when and where it occurs. Psychiatric categories, on the other hand, are necessarily historical and mutable. If these last two statements are correct, it will be hard to make a case for natural kinds in psychiatry. However, without stretching the point too far, one might argue that no scientific kinds are truly immutable. Biological kinds certainly are not. Genomes are constantly changing due to genetic drift and the pressures of natural and sexual selection. Admittedly, some species, the 'living fossils', have shown remarkable resilience. For instance, the earliest discovered fossils of the horseshoe crab date from 450 million years ago. But in other species, such as the finches of the Galápagos Islands, evolutionary change has been witnessed in real time. The problem this raises for any concept of biological species is that categorical breaks in the historical evolution of a species would appear to be arbitrary.[35] Species A evolves into species B, but at what point in time does A end and B begin? The same difficulty must apply to human mental disorders, which are materially dependent on the human genome and subject to the same (or more rapid) processes of change.

One way to deal with the problem of temporality would be to distinguish between strong natural kinds (e.g. in chemistry) and weaker, mutable kinds (in the life sciences). However, chemical kinds are not in fact immutable.[36] A consensus in modern cosmology holds that the elements were created at some time (possibly thousands of years) after the big bang. During this period the universe did not yet contain the elements of the periodic table. The elements are therefore temporally limited kinds that were created by a historically determinate chain of events. Nor is it irrational to ask whether a different chain of events might have given rise to a different set of subatomic particles and elements. All we can say for certain is that within the parameters of the events that created *this* universe, chemical elements are (in these relative terms) immutable natural kinds. Conversely, to describe chemical elements as immutable natural kinds is to assume that there is a stable, big bang-created universe to house them.

---

[35] David L. Hull, 'The Effect of Essentialism on Taxonomy – Two Thousand Years of Stasis', *British Journal for the Philosophy of Science* 15 (1965), 314–26, and 16 (1965), 1–18.

[36] Peter Zachar, 'Psychiatry, Scientific Laws and Realism About Entities', in Kenneth S. Kendler and Josef Parnas (eds.), *Philosophical Issues in Psychiatry: Explanation, Phenomenology, and Nosology* (Baltimore, MD: Johns Hopkins University Press, 2008), 39–47 (at pp. 39–42).

Similar arguments can be made for biological species – for instance, Richard Boyd's proposal of 'homeostatic property cluster kinds' (HPCKs).[37] Like Dupré, Boyd thinks that no single biological property is essential for membership of a species. A species would qualify as an HPCK by sharing a cluster of stable similarities. The requirement for HPCKhood is merely that the similarities among the instances of a kind must be sufficiently stable to allow a better than average chance of correctly inferring various other properties of the kind. If an animal has prominent canine teeth, a wet nose, and an ability to bark, we can infer fairly reliably that it will have a strong sense of smell and a propensity to wag its tail. The chief difference between Boyd's and Dupré's accounts is that Boyd builds a causal element into his concept of a natural kind. The cluster of properties that constitutes an HPCK remains stable because of homeostatic mechanisms – that is, mechanisms that regulate properties and thus prevent them from diverging too far from a norm. In the case of a biological species these mechanisms would include genetic exchange between the members of the species through breeding, and the selection pressures that arise from inhabiting a shared environment. If we assume that these pressures remain relatively stable, as in our big bang-created universe, the homeostatic mechanisms will ensure that any species inhabiting the niche will also remain relatively stable.

7   Human kinds

Animal behaviour, though culturally variable, is also genetically determined.[38] Behaviour is part of an animal's 'extended phenotype', in Richard Dawkins's phrase.[39] If an animal's anatomy and physiology are phenotypic expressions of its genotype, its behaviour is no less so. Since animal behaviour includes emotions and their expression, we have the basis for an argument that emotions are biological natural kinds. And if emotions are natural kinds, we have stronger grounds for thinking that mental disorders are natural kinds.

In *The Expression of the Emotions in Man and Animals* (1872), Darwin argued that some human emotions, such as fear in response to a threat, are

---

[37] Richard Boyd, 'Realism, Anti-Foundationalism and the Enthusiasm for Natural Kinds', *Philosophical Studies* 61 (1991), 127–48, and 'Homeostasis, Species, and Higher Taxa', in Robert A. Wilson (ed.), *Species: New Interdisciplinary Essays* (Cambridge, MA: MIT Press, 1999), 141–85.

[38] On cultural variability in primate behaviour, see Christophe Boesch, *Wild Cultures: A Comparison Between Chimpanzee and Human Cultures* (Cambridge University Press, 2012).

[39] Richard Dawkins, *The Extended Phenotype: The Long Reach of the Gene* (Oxford University Press, 1999).

universal.[40] Found in all human populations, these emotions work via subconscious systems – hormonal and neurological, muscular-skeletal, and expressive. In these emotional systems we can trace a direct path leading from the experience of a threat to the subconscious generation of a response and thence to the visible expression of an emotion. This direct path has several evolutionary benefits, the most obvious of which are the speed and consistency of the responses it generates. Speed of response is vital in life or death situations; consistency of response is advantageous in social situations. Researchers in this Darwinian tradition, most prominently Paul Ekman, have identified a small set of emotions that function in this manner and are considered to be evolutionarily evolved response mechanisms. Silvan Tomkins labelled these the 'affect programs'.[41] The set is generally held to comprise six emotions: happiness, sadness, fear, anger, surprise, and disgust. Each has its own particular triggers, mechanisms, and gestural and facial expressions. These properties of the affect programmes appear to be uniform across all human populations. Using Boyd's version of natural kinds, Paul Griffiths has argued that the affect programmes can be classified as HPCKs.[42]

For strategic reasons Griffiths limits the range of natural kind emotions to the small set of six affect programmes. Understandably he wants to focus attention on emotions that have been the subject of extensive scientific research. The strategy also enables him to exclude the complex, messy, and less well understood 'higher' emotions, which may be more culturally variable. The affect programmes, by contrast, are held to be 'cognitively impenetrable'.[43] They are impervious to thought; no effort of reflection by us could change the way they function. We might be able to train ourselves to limit their impact on us, but we cannot change the *manner* in which they function. The higher emotions, by contrast, are cognitively penetrable. After reflecting on my jealousy, I may experience it in a quite different way.

Arguably, Griffiths's strategy of limitation is damaging and unnecessary. It would certainly prove hard to accommodate depression and melancholia within Griffiths's theory, as these experiences obviously are

---

[40] Charles Darwin, *The Expression of the Emotions in Man and Animals*, with introduction, notes and commentaries by Paul Ekman (London: HarperCollins, 1998).

[41] Silvan S. Tomkins, *Affect, Imagery, and Consciousness*, 4 vols. (New York: Springer, 1962–92). See also Paul Ekman, *Emotions Revealed: Understanding Faces and Feelings* (London: Weidenfeld & Nicholson, 2003).

[42] Paul Griffiths, *What Emotions Really Are: The Problem of Psychological Categories* (University of Chicago Press, 1997), 188.

[43] On cognitive penetrability, see Z. W. Pylyshyn, *Computation and Cognition* (Cambridge, MA: MIT Press, 1984).

cognitively penetrable. Their cognitive content – e.g. pessimism or loss of self-worth – can be modified by reflection. Indeed, this is precisely the rationale of some forms of psychotherapy such as cognitive behavioural therapy (CBT). Through a course of CBT patients can learn to turn their pessimism or self-hatred into more productive thoughts. Their high degree of cognitive content is also likely to make melancholia and depression highly culturally variable. In particular, culturally specific notions of the self are likely to generate their own specific forms of melancholia or depression. (The idea that the cultural specificity of melancholia is largely a product of Western notions of the self is one of the central arguments of this book.) Thus, whereas the homeostatic mechanisms regulating the affect programmes would be purely evolutionary (sharing of genetic material, and common pressures of environmental and sexual selection), the mechanisms regulating the higher mental disorders such as melancholia and depression would include socio-cultural factors. One important corollary of the argument for mental disorders as natural kinds is that they must be dependent on a shared socio-cultural experience. A major part of the argument of this book is concerned with identifying what this shared socio-cultural experience is.

Griffiths's exclusion of the cognitively penetrable higher emotions may also be unnecessary. Advocates of psychiatric natural kinds face the objection that the *kind*ness of natural kinds ought to be unaffected by human actions. In what sense are natural kinds *natural* if humans can alter them? A similar objection has been made to biological natural kinds: biological species are subject to the influence of human action, and they are subject to human action in ways that materially affect their genetic make-up. All manner of organisms have had their behaviour altered by human contact, whether they are domesticated animals bred by humans, wild animals cohabiting with humans, or organisms suffering direct attack or collateral damage from man-made chemicals. And, of course, all of these species have to contend with the changes to the planet's environment wrought by humans.

Similar considerations apply to psychiatry. Of course, Foucault, Hacking, and Borch-Jakobsen are right to argue that psychiatric kinds exist in a man-made environment. Despite the attempts of evolutionary psychologists to argue that human minds (and therefore psychopathologies) are essentially the products of a stable and ahistorical 'environment of evolutionary adaptedness',[44] human mental states have, of course, been subject to the complex impact of social existence as far back as the

---

[44] Leda Cosmides and John Tooby, 'Toward an Evolutionary Taxonomy of Treatable Conditions', *Journal of Abnormal Psychology* 108 (1999), 453–64.

historical record goes, and almost certainly much further. The various epochal changes in human society – from the development of animal husbandry, through agriculture, urbanization, and trade, to the advent of the industrial and communications ages – can be expected to have wrought changes in the nature of mental illness to at least the same extent as humans have changed non-human organisms.

Earlier I defined a natural kind as something whose *kind*ness was unaffected by human action. That clearly needs to be qualified. Even some paradigmatically natural kinds would not exist without human action. Selective breeding has created new species and new kinds of domesticated animals. Even though these are the product of human action, we rightly accept them as natural kinds. Their *kind*ness is not intrinsically different from that of non-domesticated species. When a biologist differentiates one species from another, it makes no *biological* difference whether the two species are domesticated or wild: the biological facts that make a cocker spaniel different from a Siamese cat are not of a different order from the facts that make a wolf different from a tiger.

Are there any fundamental differences between these man-made biological natural kinds and psychiatric kinds? Some philosophers have argued that there are. As Immanuel Kant pointed out, if we think of physics as the paradigmatic science, then psychology has only a dubious claim to the status of a science. Kant's argument was that the objects of psychology, unlike those of physics, are *always* affected by the scientist's actions and interests. The evidence used in psychological research is either (a) subjectively reported or (b) objectively observed. If it is (a) subjectively reported, the process of self-observation and report affects the mind being observed: in observing ourselves we are altering the very behaviour we profess to be observing. If the evidence is (b) objectively observed, the persons being observed will know they are being observed, and this will affect their behaviour.[45]

Kant's strictures on the status of psychology have been developed further by Ian Hacking. Hacking has focused on the history of multiple-personality disorder, but his findings could equally apply to depression. In the process of describing and classifying human minds, psychiatry creates feedback – for instance, in the form of the class 'depression' – which affects the patients to whom it is applied. During or after diagnosis, patients may be made aware of features of the class depression of which they were previously unaware, and may subsequently behave in ways

[45] See the account of Kant's attitude to psychology in Matthew Bell, *The German Tradition of Psychology in Literature and Thought, 1700–1840* (Cambridge University Press, 2005), 145–7.

which react to the diagnosis. The classification of depression may thus bring into being a new class of people with a subtly different form of depressive disorder. To complete Hacking's argument, the behaviour of this new class of people would then feed back into the process of classification via subsequent research, and the diagnosis would change accordingly. Hacking has named these recursive effects 'looping' effects. He concludes that psychiatric kinds, for which he coins the term 'human kinds', are fundamentally different from natural kinds.[46]

Hacking's notion of a distinct class of human kinds has been criticized for failing to establish a fundamental difference between human and natural kinds. Rachel Cooper and Muhammad Ali Khalidi have argued that all Hacking has done is to show that psychiatric taxa are subject to the same sorts of interactions with humans as, say, the taxa of domesticated animals are.[47] As Cooper points out, the keystone of Hacking's argument concerns our awareness of being classified. Psychiatric patients are not just affected (whether directly or indirectly) by the actions of psychiatrists; the key is that they are *aware* of being so affected. But why is awareness fundamental? One argument might be that this awareness results in inauthentic behaviour. Patients might start to pretend that they conform to the psychiatrists' expectations of them. If this inauthentic behaviour is then mistakenly interpreted by psychiatrists as symptomatic of an actual disorder, the argument for Hacking's 'human kinds' would be compelling. However, this is not Hacking's argument. In fact, Hacking argues that the changes in behaviour are authentic, not pretended.[48] So there seems to be no reason to distinguish between looping effects in 'human kinds' and in biological natural kinds.

8   Socially constructed natural kinds

If there is no reason in principle to distinguish Hacking's human kinds from, say, Boyd's HPCKs, the fact of human impact on mental disorders is not a reason to disallow psychiatric kinds. We would have to grant that psychiatric kinds are historical and mutable. But we have already acknowledged the historical nature of all natural kinds, including the chemical elements. Our definition of a natural kind does not depend on its supposed historical immutability, but on the thought that all natural kinds enjoy relative permanence within the context of their own homeostatic

---

[46] Ian Hacking, *The Social Construction of What?* (Cambridge, MA: Harvard University Press, 1999), ch. 4.
[47] Cooper, 'Why Hacking Is Wrong', 73–85; Khalidi, 'Interactive Kinds', 335–60.
[48] Cooper, 'Why Hacking Is Wrong', 79.

systems, whether they are chemical kinds (e.g. elements), astronomical kinds (galaxies), geological kinds (rock formations), biological kinds (species), psychological kinds (affects), or psychiatric kinds (mental disorders). Human social formations obviously play a very significant role in the homeostasis of psychiatric kinds, as they do for many biological species, whether domestic animals or wild animals affected by human action.

A significant advantage of this reasoning is that it allows for kinds to be natural and at the same time socially constructed. By 'socially constructed' I mean that mental disorders are to some extent socially constructed facts. Hacking's 1998 study *Mad Travellers: Reflections on the Reality of Transient Mental Illnesses* provides a good example of a socially constructed mental disorder. Hacking's subject matter is the appearance and disappearance of the psychiatric diagnosis of *fugue* (also known as 'ambulatory automatism'). Beginning around 1890 and lasting for two or three decades, psychiatrists found cases of people (almost exclusively men) who would compulsively undertake long journeys on foot, with no sense of why they were travelling and often no sense of their own identity. Hacking classifies *fugue* as a 'transient mental illness', by which he means 'an illness that appears at a time, in a place, and later fades away':

It may spread from place to place and reappear from time to time. It may be selective for social class and gender, preferring poor women or rich men. I do not mean that it comes and goes in this or that patient, but that this type of madness exists only at certain times and places.[49]

In order to explain why the diagnosis 'exists only at certain times', Hacking invokes a set of four vectors, as he terms them, which allowed the phenomenon to become prominent. First, fugue fitted into an available space in the medical taxonomy of the time. Second, it captured the public imagination because it seemed to sit ambiguously between two cultural phenomena that were of urgent interest: romantic tourism and 'criminal' vagrancy. Third, it was visible and noteworthy behaviour, the sort of thing that was likely to be picked up. And fourth, it appeared to provide some sort of release from social pressures for those who experienced it. This set of vectors, Hacking argues, coalesced only for a brief period. During this window, the phenomenon and diagnosis of fugue made sense. Once the window closed, interest in fugue waned: the number of cases dwindled, and the few fugue-like cases that sporadically appeared were diagnosed under other categories.

The socially constructed component of fugue obviously reaches deep down into the disorder's structure. Fugue occurred in a culture in which

---

[49] Hacking, *Mad Travellers*, 1.

vagrancy was common and of pressing concern. But fugue was definitely a *transient* mental illness; it existed only for a short time, a mere mayfly in comparison to the Methuselah melancholia. Considering these two facts about fugue, that it was short-lived and deeply socially constructed, we might formulate the following hypothesis. A mental disorder that is socially constructed in its deep structure is likely to be relatively unstable, as social formations are themselves volatile. By contrast, a mental disorder that is mainly organic and has only superficial socially constructed components will be relatively long-lived. Indeed, the relative stability of a disorder over historical time might even function as a heuristic for determining whether it is predominantly organic or socially constructed.

If this hypothesis were correct, we might expect melancholia, a disorder of great longevity, to be predominantly organic. Recall, however, that we have earlier decided that melancholia must be highly cognitively penetrable and therefore prone to social influences. Melancholia thus appears to disconfirm our hypothesis: it is a mental disorder that is substantially socially constructed and yet at the same time very stable. One way to deal with this difficulty would be to revise our intuition that social causes are normally relatively unstable and of short duration. Indeed, Murphy argues that certain forms or combinations of social vectors might be relatively stable:

The persistence of a disorder in relatively unchanged form across the generations does not show that it is not partly a cultural product. If a niche comes into existence because of the coalescence of vectors, why should it not persist? If the vectors fall into a stable configuration robust enough to withstand cultural changes then the niche may endure indefinitely.[50]

In other words, there may be social vectors that are semi-permanent, and these vectors might combine to form a stable niche in which a particular mental disorder might itself become semi-permanent, despite being deeply cognitively penetrable.

A further problem in the historiography of melancholia, as we will see in Chapter 5, is that the factors usually adduced to explain the emergence of melancholia – the rise of individualism, the experience of religious schism, the emergence of early capitalism – either do not reach a sufficiently high standard of robustness, in Murphy's terms, or are not present in the historical period that is in need of explanation. In order to explain the longevity of melancholia we need to find a more robust set of vectors that has extended right across the period from Hippocrates to the modern day. In the following chapters, I propose such an account of the persistence of

---

[50] Murphy, *Psychiatry in the Scientific Image*, 268.

melancholia. It will depend on two vectors. These are (a) a commitment to a kind-based conception of mental medicine involving continuous empirical testing and theoretical debate, and (b) what I will call a culture of self-consciousness. In the West both of these vectors originated in Ancient Greece during the hundred or so years before the first surviving references to melancholia in the Hippocratic writings.[51] My argument is that melancholia could become prominent and widely used only when a realist mental medicine and a culture of self-consciousness had become embedded in fifth-century BC Greece, and that melancholia's continuing prominence within Western culture and latterly the spread of depression to many parts of the world depend upon these same vectors. Before the emergence of a realist mental medicine and a culture of self-consciousness in Ancient Greece, there was no melancholia. Cases resembling melancholia can be found before the fifth century BC, notably in the Old Testament and the Gilgamesh epic (see Chapter 1). But there is no evidence that these earlier cases were subject to sustained medical analysis or that they had any wider cultural resonance. In other words, before Hippocrates, there is no evidence of a stable and widespread syndrome resembling melancholia, no evidence of a *disorder* of melancholia. The manner in which the earliest Hippocratic text talks about melancholia does make it seem likely that the disease of melancholia predated this text, but if writers before Hippocrates referred to melancholia, their works are no longer extant and we know nothing about them.[52] Before Hippocrates, there are only isolated cases of profound, melancholia-like sadness. All this changed after the emergence of a realist mental medicine and a culture of self-consciousness in Ancient Greece: the disorder of melancholia was conceptualized, became a more or less stable presence in Western medicine and culture, and, with exceptions that will need to be explained by the model, has remained so ever since.

9   Scientific medicine

What was it about Ancient Greek medicine that enabled it to bring the disorder melancholia into being? A more detailed answer to this question is set out in Chapters 1 and 2. It turns out to be a fairly complex answer, not least because Ancient Greek medicine was more complex and less

---

[51] Compare the similar argument in Allen Thiher, *Revels in Madness: Insanity in Medicine and Literature* (Ann Arbor, MI: University of Michigan Press, 1999), 11.

[52] Jacques Jouanna, 'At the Roots of Melancholy: Is Greek Medicine Melancholic?', in Jouanna, *Greek Medicine from Hippocrates to Galen: Selected Papers* (Leiden: Brill, 2012), 229–60 (at pp. 232–3).

monolithic than many later medical writers and historians have supposed. Indeed, this very complexity is part of what made Ancient Greek medicine unique among ancient medical systems, and uniquely productive. I will confine myself here to a few general remarks about the scientific character of Greek medicine and what distinguishes it from other systems with which it bears comparison (notably ancient Egyptian and Chinese medicine).

First, much of what made Greek medicine distinctive was shared with early Greek science (or natural philosophy, as it is more accurately termed) in general. Although the Hippocratic school of medicine seems to have had an uneasy relationship with natural philosophy, what the Hippocratics had in common with the natural philosophers is arguably more important than any differences between them. For instance, early Greek natural philosophers sought to give accounts of the physical world in terms of classes of phenomena. The Milesian philosophers (Thales, Anaximander, and Anaximenes) were more interested in kinds than particulars.[53] The same can be said of the Hippocratics. Hippocratic medicine understood symptoms as signs (sēmata) of underlying disorders. The particular signs were significant only insofar as they indicated the presence of a kind of illness. The author of the Hippocratic *On Regimen in Acute Diseases* stresses how important this methodology is. Whereas a patient may be tempted to blame his disease on whatever cause lies close to hand, the Hippocratic doctor will be able to distinguish 'between causal and merely concomitant factors'.[54] Thus the Hippocratics espoused a kind of realism about causal mechanisms whereby visible symptoms were produced by changes in underlying physiology. A symptom such as dysphoria was taken to be a visible sign of a commonly experienced underlying process. It is only by virtue of this concern with classes, or more specifically with grouping symptoms into disease constructs, that a diagnosis like melancholia could come about.

Second, it is implicit in this methodology that there must be close empirical observation of symptoms. While there has been much debate about the degree to which Ancient Greek natural philosophers and physicians engaged in empirical research,[55] and while it is undeniably true that Greek medicine often presented a highly rationalistic picture of bodies and illnesses (see Chapter 1, section 5, and Chapter 3, section 3), empirical observation did play an important role in Hippocratic medicine and in

[53] G. E. R. Lloyd, *Early Greek Science: Thales to Aristotle* (London: Chatto & Windus, 1970), 9.
[54] G. E. R. Lloyd, *Magic, Reason and Experience: Studies in the Origin and Development of Greek Science* (Cambridge University Press, 1979), 54.
[55] *Ibid.*, 126–9.

the Hippocratics' image of their own practice. The four books of the Hippocratic *Epidemics* are collections of detailed case histories. (We encountered some of these cases in section 1 of this Introduction.) Disease constructs in Hippocratic medicine were based partly on presuppositions about the constitution of bodies and partly on observation of empirical regularities. Indeed, it is precisely these regularities that enable Jackson to argue for continuity between melancholia and depression.

Third, Greek natural philosophy and medicine were by no means monolithic. Significant differences existed between different thinkers and schools, and these differences were played out in constant and lively theoretical debate. Indeed, one might argue that the very existence of Greek natural philosophy and medicine, or at least the kind of naturalistic medicine practised by the Hippocratics, was premised on theoretical debate. Natural philosophy distinguished itself from traditional, religious, and folk explanations for natural phenomena. Likewise Hippocratic medicine differentiated itself from folk medicine and the 'temple medicine' of the greater and lesser shrines to Asclepius, Apollo, and the other gods and heroes associated with healing. One of the key theoretical moves in Milesian natural philosophy was not to let the gods into explanations.[56] Even though the natural philosophers and physicians often did believe that the physical universe was divine in origin, their explanations tended not to rely on local acts of divine intervention. And repeatedly, scientific and medical writers criticized traditional religious explanations for natural phenomena. For instance, the author of *On the Sacred Disease* is concerned to show that epilepsy does not have a specifically divine character: '[The "Sacred Disease"] is not, in my opinion, any more divine or more sacred than other diseases but has a natural cause.'[57] As important as this secular tendency no doubt was, what is more significant for our purposes is the environment of debate in which such statements were possible. All this allowed a degree of theoretical diversity which, say, Chinese medicine did not have.[58]

The concern with kinds rather than particulars, the relatively high standing of empirical observation, and the theoretical diversity of Greek natural philosophy and medicine formed a virtuous triangle. To define natural kinds, the Greeks needed to observe empirical regularities, but also to engage in debates about different versions of kinds. Empirical

---

[56] Benjamin Farrington, *Greek Science* (Nottingham: Spokesman, 1980), 37.

[57] Hippocrates, *The Sacred Disease*, i, in *Hippocrates I*, 139. See also Lloyd, *Early Greek Science*, 54.

[58] G. E. R. Lloyd and Nathan Sivin, *The Way and the Word: Science and Medicine in Early China and Greece* (New Haven, CT: Yale University Press, 2002), 249.

observation was motivated by the search for kinds, and theoretical debate kept it honest. And meaningful scientific debate was made more productive by a commitment to talking about kinds and grounding this talk in observation. It was on the basis of this virtuous triangle that medical kinds such as melancholia could develop and become stable, even if still contested.

10   Self-consciousness

Jackie Pigeaud has argued that the ancient experience of melancholia involved a heightened focus on the self. This was partly because melancholia raised the problem of mind–body relations in an especially acute form. As we will see in Chapter 2, the causes and symptoms of melancholia might be either physical or psychological, and in most cases they were both. The course of the disease comprised episodes of both physical and mental discomfort, sometimes in parallel, sometimes in sequence. This could provoke a strong compulsion to worry about how the mental and physical aspects of the disease related to one another and hence about mind–body relations more generally. In addition, melancholics tended to become solitary, and so they might be given to reflect on their isolation from society and on their own individuality. Pigeaud tentatively suggests a link between this heightened sense of self and philosophy: '[Mélancolie] est, en quelque sorte, si l'on veut pousser un peu les choses, maladie et apprentissage naturel de la philosophie, au sens où dans cette maladie l'homme doit apprendre à guérir sa peur de la mort et sa crainte d'autrui.'[59] Melancholia is a 'malaise comme instrument de connaissance'.[60] Pigeaud's case for a link between melancholia and self-consciousness seems persuasive; the case for the philosophical nature of this link less so. If Pigeaud means that cures for melancholia could take a philosophical form, the case is strong. But cures for melancholia were not always or even predominantly philosophical. Religious cures have also been common.[61] Most of the cures prescribed by ancient medics were purely physical (diet, exercise, etc.). Of the psychological cures, most were resolutely practical: avoid solitude, engage in conversation, listen to music, have sex. As for Pigeaud's tentative proposal that ancient melancholia had some intrinsic philosophical content, the evidence is less strong. Several ancient medical writers across quite a broad front did list a tendency to meditation among

---

[59] Pigeaud, '*Prolégomènes*', 506.
[60] Jackie Pigeaud, *Melancholia: Le malaise de l'individu* (Paris: Payot & Rivages, 2008), 24.
[61] See Jeremy Schmidt, *Melancholy and the Care of the Soul: Religion, Moral Philosophy and Madness in Early Modern England* (Aldershot: Ashgate, 2007).

melancholia's symptoms, but in doing so they did not connect melancholia with philosophical thinking. Other writers outside medicine proper did so. There was an ancient tradition of finding philosophical significance in melancholia, but it was very narrow and limited to two rather strange texts. One, the pseudo-Aristotelian *Problems* XXX/1, begins with the bizarre claim that all poets, philosophers, statesmen, and heroes have been melancholics. Whoever wrote this text was evidently not a physician, and the definition of melancholia it uses is at variance with the Hippocratic definition.[62] The other text is a fanciful exchange of fictional letters, probably from the first century BC, concerning the supposed melancholia of the philosopher Democritus.[63] Aside from these two odd texts, all ancient philosophers who wrote about melancholia were concerned to condemn or cure it, not to mine it for philosophical meaning.

Louis Sass has also constructed an analogy between self-consciousness and mental disorders – in this case, schizophrenia. In Sass's view, schizophrenics have an extreme compulsion to think solipsistically. Their talk can be interpreted as alternating between two beliefs: that the world is nothing but the self, and that the self is nothing but the world. Sass thinks that these two conjoined positions are analogous to Wittgenstein's diagnosis of the history of Western philosophy.[64] Using the infamous Schreber case as evidence, Sass argues that schizophrenia pushes the absurdities of rarefied forms of modern philosophy to their twin and contradictory logical conclusions. Sass's account of schizophrenia as heightened self-consciousness has some affinities with my argument. But I think both Pigeaud and Sass try to eke too much philosophical significance out of mental disorders.[65] It is certainly true that some philosophers in the modern period have found philosophical meaning in melancholia or conditions like it. Schopenhauer, Nietzsche, and Sartre are obvious examples, and there is an argument for tracing this tradition back as far as Hume or even Petrarch, as we will see in Chapter 5. But philosophical melancholia of this kind has more to do with pessimism and scepticism than with self-consciousness. Chapter 5 will also consider some of the reasons why melancholy has proved so fertile in literature.

In other words, while I am sceptical about the evidence that has been presented for the philosophical character of mental disorders, I would like to leave open the possibility that melancholy self-consciousness can in

---

[62] Jouanna, 'At the Roots of Melancholy', 243.   [63] See Pigeaud, '*Prolégomènes*', 505–6.
[64] Louis A. Sass, *The Paradoxes of Delusion: Wittgenstein, Schreber, and the Schizophrenic Mind* (Ithaca, NY: Cornell University Press, 1994), 69.
[65] See the critique of Sass in Rupert Read, 'On Approaching Schizophrenia Through Wittgenstein', *Philosophical Psychology* 14 (2001), 449–75.

some instances have a philosophical dimension. But my primary definition
of self-consciousness will not be a philosophical one. By self-consciousness
I mean a socially or culturally approved habit of talking about one's own
mental and emotional states. The vector of self-consciousness is a socio-
cultural fact, not a philosophical idea, and is therefore not in need of a
philosophical definition. It may be that at some times and in some places
the reasons for valuing self-consciousness have included philosophical
ideas, such as Socrates' dictum that 'the unexamined life is not worth living'
or Descartes's notion of consciousness as a kind of internal theatre. Where
such powerful philosophical notions of self-consciousness are found,
evidence of a broader *culture* of self-consciousness will be found too. But
that broader culture of self-consciousness is not necessarily dependent on
strong philosophical notions of the Socratic or Cartesian kind. The philosophical justification of self-consciousness is only one of several possible
sources of justification. Another source of justification, arguably more
important in historical terms, has been religion, in particular early modern
Protestantism. Cultural fashions have also sanctioned self-consciousness,
notably eighteenth-century sensibility and romanticism.

If self-consciousness is not primarily a philosophical idea, what is it?
I believe the best way to define self-consciousness for the purposes of this
discussion is in the fairly neutral and modest terms of cognitive and social
psychology. I have in mind psychological concepts such as 'self-focused
attention'. Rick Ingram defines self-focused attention as 'an awareness of
self-referent, internally generated information that stands in contrast to
an awareness of externally generated information derived through sensory
receptors'.[66] This concept is broadly compatible with, though less specific
and therefore more widely applicable than, comparable philosophical
notions of self-consciousness. It should be assumed in the following
chapters that when I use the term 'self-consciousness' I mean something
close to Ingram's definition of self-focused attention.

In addition to its philosophical neutrality, self-focused attention has
the advantage of belonging to the cognitive psychology of melancholia
and depression. Pigeaud has argued that melancholia causes sufferers
to reflect on their selfhood.[67] It is implicit in the DSM-5 construction
of major depressive disorder that depression involves self-focus. One of
DSM's primary symptoms of depression is excessive or inappropriate

---

[66] Rick E. Ingram, 'Self-Focused Attention in Clinical Disorders: Review and a Conceptual
Model', *Psychological Bulletin* 107 (1990), 156–76 (at p. 156).

[67] 'La mélancolie engage, plus que d'autres maladies que, pour faire vite, nous appellerons
psychiques, la relation de l'âme et du corps, et la relation de l'individu avec autrui … La
mélancolie est donc une maladie qui met en question la relation de soi avec soi-même',
Pigeaud, '*Prolégomènes*', 506.

guilt, and guilt contains the idea of self-blame and hence self-focus. Recent work in the cognitive psychology of depression has gone much further than DSM and has consistently shown a positive correlation between depression and a tendency to self-focus.[68] Those suffering from depression have a stronger tendency to self-focus than non-depressed people, and a strong tendency to self-focus is liable to intensify and prolong the depressive illness. Depressed people tend to show a 'self-focusing style' that involves intense focus on the self after some perceived failure; they are more likely to blame themselves for their failures than they are to give themselves credit for their successes.[69] Their attention to self can verge on a kind of 'self-absorption' that is characterized by 'excessive, sustained, and rigid attention' to the self.[70] Depressed people will often engage in 'rumination' on their own depression – in other words, 'behaviours and thoughts that focus one's attention on one's depressive symptoms and on the implications of these symptoms'.[71] And rumination is strongly associated with failure to recover from depression. Patients who compulsively ruminate are less liable to interpret positive experiences for what they are and so to lift themselves out of depression.

While the ruminative cognition of depressed people may be characterized as pathological, it should not necessarily be characterized as a deficit or lack of cognitive effort. (Indeed, rumination might arguably be better characterized as an *excess* of cognitive effort in a particular direction.) Instead of seeing melancholy cognition as a lack, in this book I see it as a *style*. One might draw an analogy with recent research on autism. Traditionally, autistic behaviour was understood as a deficit of certain cognitive abilities, such as empathy or mind-reading. But the cognitive deficit model made it hard to account for autistic savant behaviour, where autism is accompanied by prodigious skills in, say, music or art. Newer approaches recognize autistic thinking as a cognitive style marked by looser central coherence. This looser central coherence allows remarkable focus on very local matters, and this may be what lies behind autistic savant behaviour.[72] Alternatively, autistic savants may possess extremely deep memory capacity that enables them to perform exceptionally well in art, music, or mathematics, but which they find it hard to apply to social

---

[68] See the literature cited in Tom Pyszczynski and Jeff Greenberg, 'Evidence for a Depressive Self-Focusing Style', *Journal of Research in Personality* 20 (1986), 95–106 (at p. 95).

[69] Pyszczynski and Greenberg, 'Evidence', 102–5.

[70] Ingram, 'Self-Focused Attention', 173.

[71] Susan Nolen-Hoeksema, 'Responses to Depression and Their Effects on the Duration of Depressive Episodes', *Journal of Abnormal Psychology* 100 (1991), 569–82 (at p. 569).

[72] Francesca Happé, 'Autism: Cognitive Deficit or Cognitive Style?', *Trends in Cognitive Sciences* 3 (1999), 216–22.

situations.[73] By preferring *style* to *deficit*, I do not in the first place mean to remove a stigma from mental disorders (though that would be a worthy end). Rather I have two historical arguments in mind. As we will see in Chapter 4, some social, political, and historical outlooks have been strongly coloured by melancholia. Often, and mistakenly in my view, these have been portrayed as unworthy of serious consideration. Here we might compare a valuable study by Joshua Foa Dienstag of philosophical pessimism. Dienstag shows that the long and eminent tradition of pessimistic politics in the West has been shamefully neglected by historians of political thought.[74] In a similar way, melancholy political stances tend to be dismissed as weakly passive or as instances of false consciousness. My view is that these judgements are undeserved. A second point follows from the connection between melancholia and self-consciousness. Self-consciousness is a defining feature of Western culture, and melancholia has played an important role in shaping and giving expression to the way we are conscious of ourselves. One need only consider the large quantity (and high quality) of melancholy art, music, and especially literature in the West. Like autistic savant behaviour, these cultural expressions are hard to explain if melancholy cognition is understood merely as a deficit.

In other words, research into depressive self-focused attention suggests that we may be close to the mark in positing this psychological form of self-consciousness as one of the vectors responsible for melancholia and depression. The idea of self-focused attention allows us to build a bridge between our normally harmless socio-cultural vector – talk focusing on one's own mental and emotional states – and the pathological self-focusing cognitions characteristic of depressed people. Let us assume that the difference between normal self-consciousness and pathological self-focus is one of degree: pathological self-focus and normal self-consciousness are on a continuum. Just as depressive self-focused attention develops out of normal self-consciousness, we might assume that melancholia and depression, with their intense forms of self-focus, will only evolve out of a social and culture milieu that already places a high value on normal self-consciousness. The fact that a society approves of self-consciousness allows its members to develop the extreme and pathological self-focusing behaviour of melancholia.

---

[73] D. A. Treffert, 'The Savant Syndrome: An Extraordinary Condition. A Synopsis: Past, Present, Future', *Philosophical Transactions of the Royal Society of London. Series B: Biological Sciences* 364 (2009), 1351–7.

[74] Joshua Foa Dienstag, *Pessimism: Philosophy, Ethic, Spirit* (Princeton University Press, 2006).

It is important to avoid the impression that the existence of a culture that values self-consciousness is a binary or monolithic phenomenon – that it is either there or not there; and that if it is there, it is everywhere. Cultures that value self-consciousness have been historically variable in their presence, intensity, and kind. It is tempting to generalize and say that self-consciousness has been more prevalent in modernity. And one might speculate on the reasons for this: was it the rise of individualism or of capitalism or of the Protestant confessions? These arguments are considered in Chapters 4 and 5. One might also think that until recently cultures of self-consciousness have been chiefly a Western phenomenon. What is clear is that not all societies have valued or encouraged self-consciousness to the same degree. Equally, cultures of self-consciousness, where they exist, are not all of the same nature. The forms that self-consciousness takes can vary enormously, depending on prevailing cultural norms. And within a given society tensions can exist between elements that encourage self-consciousness and those that discourage it. One might think of nineteenth-century British culture with its intense sentimentality on the one hand and its stoical stiff upper lip on the other. And just because a culture develops a sophisticated philosophical capacity to reflect on the self, it does not necessarily follow that such reflection is viewed as a good. To take the example of a massive and complex tradition such as Indian Buddhism, there are within Buddhist thought sophisticated reflexive notions of self-awareness.[75] At several points in this book I draw non-Western material into the argument by way of comparison. The intention is not to suggest that Western culture possesses something, self-consciousness, that non-Western cultures lack. On the contrary, in the case of Buddhism there is overwhelming evidence of a self-focusing style of thought. However, this self-focus is generally subordinated to a higher priority, a strong belief, already present in early Buddhism, that an excessive attachment to the self is a major cause of suffering. Buddhist enlightenment can be achieved by confining one's thoughts to external impressions; anything else can cause 'thought proliferation' (*prapañca*) which leads to 'vexation and worry'.[76] Similar ideas can be found in Graeco-Roman antiquity. We have already noted the self-awareness enjoined on us by Socrates' dictum about the unexamined life, but by no means all schools of Greek philosophy viewed attention to the self as a good. The Epicureans thought that speculation divorced from external

---

[75] Matthew MacKenzie, 'Self-Awareness Without a Self: Buddhism and the Reflexivity of Awareness', *Asian Philosophy* 18 (2008), 245–66.

[76] Thomas McEvilley, *The Shape of Ancient Thought: Comparative Studies in Greek and Indian Philosophies* (New York: Allworth Press, 2002), 603.

impressions led to the harmful proliferation of empty ideas (*kenodoxia*).[77] Empty ideas are, in fact, a key symptom of melancholia. Among the 'general symptoms' of melancholia listed by the medieval physician Isḥāq ibn ʿImrān (d. AD 903/9), who wrote in Arabic, is a tendency to think about things that do not exist.[78] As Constantinus Africanus puts it in his translation of Isḥāq ibn ʿImrān, melancholics display 'thought about things that ought not to be thought about [and] perception of things that do not exist'.[79]

Having stressed the complexity and variability of cultures of self-consciousness, I must add one further reservation. This is a short book about a huge subject. It does not profess to be a detailed history of melancholia, which would have been an undertaking on an altogether different scale. What this book offers is an *outline* of a cultural and intellectual history of melancholia. Its argument is schematic. At some points I have simplified in order to clarify. This applies in particular to some of the literary and philosophical material that I consider in Chapters 3, 4, and 5. There is no detailed literary criticism or philosophical exegesis in these pages. The bibliography lists many books and articles that present such detailed analysis. This book does not replace such detailed analysis; it outlines a new perspective from which such analysis might be done.

---

[77] See David Konstan, *A Life Worthy of the Gods: The Materialist Psychology of Epicurus* (Las Vegas, NV: Parmenides, 2008), *passim* (e.g. 17).

[78] Isḥāq ibn ʿImrān, *Maqāla fiʾl-mālīḫūliyā (Abhandlung über die Melancholie)*, and Constantinus Africanus, *Libri duo de melancholia*, ed. and trans. Karl Garbers (Hamburg: Buske, 1977), 27.

[79] Constantinus Africanus, *Libri duo de melancholia*, in Isḥāq ibn ʿImrān, *Maqāla fiʾl-mālīḫūliyā*, 120.

1 Naming a disease

1 Kind history and linguistic history

What happened to melancholia in the twentieth century? By 'melancholia' I mean the term *melancholia* as a label for a nosological category. The simple answer is that in mainstream psychiatry it was replaced by depression. But things are more complex. Melancholia did not go away entirely. It remained in continuous use on the margins of psychiatry, as, for instance, in psychoanalysis. In 2008 the British psychoanalyst Darian Leader published an essay titled *The New Black: Mourning, Melancholia and Depression.*[1] Leader's title pays homage to Freud's 1917 essay 'Mourning and Melancholia', which has been the starting point for psychoanalytical investigations of melancholia ever since. However, Freud's essay is, to say the least, ambivalent about the value of melancholia as a diagnosis: at the outset Freud doubts whether melancholia is even a meaningful diagnosis.[2] This may be because the psychoanalytical system was better equipped (and was indeed expressly designed) to address the conditions that used to be known as hysteria: these were the conditions that first excited Freud's interest and gave rise to his first major theoretical breakthroughs.

Melancholia has also continued in use in mainstream psychiatry, albeit again in an oddly marginal form. Successive editions of DSM have included melancholia as a 'features specifier' of depression. For instance, in DSM-5 (2013), certain depressive disorders – major depressive episode (single or recurrent) and bipolar disorders I and II – can be specified as having a set of 'melancholic' features in addition to their usual list of symptoms. The features that count as 'melancholic' are as follows:

[1] Darian Leader, *The New Black: Mourning, Melancholia and Depression* (London: Hamish Hamilton, 2008).
[2] Sigmund Freud, 'Mourning and Melancholia', in Freud, *On Murder, Mourning and Melancholia*, trans. Shaun Whiteside (London: Penguin, 2005), 201–18 (at p. 201).

Loss of pleasure in all, or almost all, activities, lack of reactivity to usually pleasurable stimuli ... a distinct quality of depressed mood [i.e. the depressed mood is experienced as distinctly different from feeling of grief experienced after the death of a loved one], depression that is regularly worse in the morning, early morning awakening ... marked psychomotor agitation or retardation, significant anorexia or weight loss, excessive or inappropriate guilt.[3]

What is odd about the presence of melancholia in DSM is that the purpose of a features specifier is to mark out a distinctive subcategory with additional typical characteristics. So the features specified by the specifier need to be different from those of the head category. But most of the 'melancholic' features are identical to the standard symptoms of non-'melancholic' depression: there is very little substantive difference between the melancholic features and the symptoms of major depressive disorder. The sole feature of melancholic depression that is absent from major depressive disorder is melancholia's supposedly distinctive diurnal rhythm of early waking and bad mornings. The other features are identical: depressed mood, loss of pleasure, disturbed sleep patterns, inability to concentrate, weight loss, and guilt. In other words, melancholic depression describes a set of symptoms that are, with one exception, identical to depressive illness. And this points towards the paradoxical situation that melancholia finds itself in today. As a kind, melancholia is anything but marginal: its symptoms are central to the definition of depression. But as a psychiatric term or label for a nosological category, it has been reduced to a mere adjective, and an adjective that brings very little to the party.

Having largely discarded the term *melancholia*, twentieth-century psychiatrists continued to work with a disease construct, depression, that shared its core psychological symptoms with the melancholia observed by Hippocrates over 2,000 years earlier. The contrast between the history of a kind and the history of a term could hardly be more striking than in the case of *melancholia*. The former has been a history of broad continuity, the latter one of long dominance followed by marginalization and recent signs of a return. In this chapter, I investigate the history of the terms *melancholia* and *depression*. The aim will be to explain why the history of the terms has the shape it does. In order to remind us that it is the terms we are talking about, and not the kinds, I will follow the practice of placing the words *melancholia* and *depression* in italics where they refer to the terms, not the kind. The italics will disappear in Chapter 2, when we return to the history of the kind.

---

[3] DSM-5, 185.

2 Metaphors and etymology

One of Taylor and Fink's arguments for reinstating *melancholia* is that the term summons up a long and august medical 'heritage' dating back to Hippocrates.[4] It is odd to find cutting-edge science making an appeal to heritage, though here again we need to distinguish between name history and kind history. Scientists construct kinds in what Hans Reichenbach called the 'context of justification', where the only valid considerations should be empirical, methodological, and theoretical factors from within science.[5] Language operates according to quite different principles. As Saussure showed, the ways we use a word are determined by two sorts of factors: how we (here and now) choose to use the word in relation to other words (*cold* in relation to *freezing, cool, warm*, etc.), and the traditions of usage stretching back through the history of the language (English *cold* and German *kalt* descend from a common Germanic ancestor). In this latter sense, usage is the heir of history. Despite its evident irrationality, we cannot and would not want to free ourselves from the history of our language. Its history is in large part responsible for a language's internal structure, without which we would have chaos and madness. (This is why opponents of spelling reform, who insist that etymology should continue to influence spelling and who are often caricatured as conservative pedants for doing so, actually have strong arguments on their side.) And that is why usage is the heir of history and not its prisoner. History is a very wealthy and munificent parent. But in a case such as *melancholia* or *depression*, the richness of history can make the decision a complex one.

Despite its rich historical heritage, the return of *melancholia* is not easy to explain. Over the last hundred years we have grown comfortable with the word *depression*. It denotes a set of feelings and behaviours we can easily observe, and it helpfully conveys these through the metaphor of being pressed or weighed down. And disregarding for a moment the many contentious issues in recent research into depression, the clinical use of the term *depression* is actually quite close to its everyday use. The DSM-5 specification for major depressive episode includes symptoms that are naturally and aptly covered by the word *depression*: low mood, feelings of sadness or emptiness, diminished interest or pleasure in otherwise pleasurable activities, fatigue or loss of energy, feelings of worthlessness or excessive guilt, diminished ability to think or concentrate, and recurrent thoughts of death. The label is a natural fit for a mind weighed down by

---

[4] Taylor and Fink, *Melancholia*, 45.
[5] Hans Reichenbach, 'On Probability and Induction', *Philosophy of Science* 5 (1938), 21–45.

the world and itself. In the word *depression* there is a reassuring continuum between the realms of science and everyday experience.

The word *melancholia* has no such advantages. There is nothing reassuringly metaphorical about it. It is far less intuitive than *depression*. In linguistic terms, it is foreign. Etymologically, it descends from Ancient Greek via Latin. Aside from its anglicized form *melancholy* and the adjective *melancholic*, it has no widely used cognates. By contrast, *depression* belongs to a large family of semantically related words that are in everyday use. These include the verb *depress* and many other words formed with -*press*, such as *oppress* and *repress*. Not least thanks to its large number of relatives, *depression* helpfully connects the mental disorder to a set of commonly verbalized experiences.

In their proposal to rehabilitate *melancholia*, Taylor and Fink use the Latinized Greek form *melancholia*, not the anglicized *melancholy*, no doubt because of an institutional reflex. One function of medicine's Latinized Greek terminology is to fix a linguistic boundary between medical and normal usage. Assuming we observe the boundary, we can be clear whether we are talking about a disorder recognized by medical science or we are expressing everyday (and scientifically worthless) folk knowledge. Aside from this fairly trivial fact of institutional sociology, in the case of *melancholia/melancholy* there are understandable reasons for not wanting to blur the line between medical knowledge (*melancholia*) and 'folk' knowledge (*melancholy*). *Melancholy* in today's English usage suggests a range of unserious, medically insignificant behaviours: pensiveness, wistfulness, self-indulgence, and a sadness that is knowing and perhaps even moderately pleasurable. In using the word *melancholy* of yourself, you would be portraying yourself as a literary sort, fond of old-fashioned language, perhaps even living somewhere in the past, when people did indeed really suffer from melancholy (or could plausibly claim to), a past in which depression was unknown as a medical disorder, and when indeed medicine itself was a more gentlemanly occupation.[6] And you would most certainly distinguish your own state from that of drab, common-or-garden depression. With your melancholy gloom would come discernment, elevation above the masses, and not a little pretentiousness.

3   Tradition

One powerful antirealist argument often used in the historiography of melancholia is that *melancholia* has changed its meaning so much over

---

[6] Michael Bywater, *Lost Worlds: What Have We Lost, and Where Did It Go?* (Cambridge: Granta, 2004), 176–7.

2,500 years that it cannot be understood as a single concept. How can we defend the reality of mental disorders when the usage of their labels has undergone such dramatic change?

In his *Life of Theseus* Plutarch tells the story of the preservation of the ship in which Theseus sailed to Crete to rescue the youth of Athens from the Minotaur:

> The ship on which Theseus sailed with the youths and returned in safety, the thirty-oared galley, was preserved by the Athenians down to the time of Demetrius Phalereus [*c.* 350–*c.* 280 BC]. They took away the old timbers from time to time, and put new and sound ones in their places, so that the vessel became a standing illustration for the philosophers in the mooted question of growth, some declaring that it remained the same, others that it was not the same vessel.[7]

The paradox of Theseus' ship is usually cited in philosophical discussions of identity, but it can also shed light on a tradition like that of melancholia. Modern discussions of the idea of tradition rightly stress that any intervention in a tradition involves remaking the tradition. One might argue that, even if only to the minimal extent of replacing a rotten plank with an identical new one, intervening in a tradition is a creative act: it amounts to remaking the ship. On the other hand, the emphasis on creativity – the word *intervention* is loaded – can tend to underestimate the extent to which tradition is mere conservation. I say *mere* conservation, though in fact conservation for the sake of conservation contains its own ideological presuppositions. Even if the effect is only to conserve, in most cases conservation happens because the conserved object has a use value, which may be ideological.

So it was with Theseus' famous ship. Originally just a means of conveyance for Theseus and the Athenian youths he brought home to safety, over time the ship became a symbol of Athens's identity. The ship represented Athens's stake in the heroic mythical past and therefore its claim to dine at the top table of Greek city states. This is where the philosophers' debate about the identity of the ship comes in. Some philosophers reasoned that the ship was no longer the same ship. Their antagonists, in claiming that the ship *was* still Theseus' ship, reduced its historical and material multiplicity – the many actions of the shipwrights, the sources of the new planks, the different molecular structure of the various species of wood – to a single idea: the virtue of the Athenian city state embodied therein. And so it is with tradition. The many of history is reduced to the one of ideology.

---

[7] *Theseus*, xxiii, in Plutarch, *Lives I*, trans. by Bernadotte Perrin, Loeb Classical Library (London: Heinemann, 1914), 49.

To return to melancholia, the many actions and meanings involved in the remaking and sustaining of the tradition of melancholia across 2,000 years are largely useless for today's medical purposes. The Graeco-Roman theory of the humours has no value for Taylor and Fink, whose purpose is to reduce melancholia to a simpler, more serviceable thing. Similarly, when depression took the place of melancholia as the head category for this psychiatric kind, the result was a useful simplification. And this process of simplification is not just a feature of modern interventions in the tradition. Repeatedly in the long history of melancholia we encounter simplifications of meaning motivated by the uses of the moment. All who add to the tradition want to make their own clear and coherent picture of the disorder, guided, of course, by whatever medical paradigms pertain at the time.

It might seem that the realism outlined in the Introduction places us in a similar position to Taylor and Fink, insofar as realism commits us to highlight those parts of the tradition for which reality can plausibly be claimed. Realism is bound to be more interested in the real than the unreal. The part of the tradition that I privilege in this book is the core psychology of melancholia. In Graeco-Roman medicine there seems to be agreement that, whatever else it was, melancholia had to display the psychological symptoms of fear and sadness. Often these were qualified by the further requirements that the fear and sadness be of long duration or have no evident cause. So in the Hippocratic *Aphorisms* we find this definition: 'Fear and depression that is prolonged means melancholia.'[8] In *On the Affected Parts* Galen confirms that while melancholia was very varied in its manifestations, fear and sadness formed its indispensable core: 'Hippocrates seems to have been right to reduce under two headings the symptoms of melancholics: fear and sadness.'[9] The justification for privileging this core psychology is threefold. First, the core psychology belongs to the earliest accounts of melancholia in the Hippocratic corpus. Over time melancholia became associated with a great number of other phenomena and ideas, but these were later embellishments. So the core psychology has historical priority. Second, from Hippocrates to Freud and beyond, the core psychology has remained remarkably consistent, as Jackson has shown. The core psychology has continued to be formulated in essentially the same terms for over 2,000 years. Third, as a nosological category melancholia owes its continuous (or nearly continuous) presence in

---

[8] Hippocrates, *Aphorisms*, 6, 23, in *Hippocrates IV*, trans. W. H. S. Jones, Loeb Classical Library (London: Heinemann, 1979), 185.

[9] Galen, *De locis affectis*, 3, 10, cited in Jouanna, 'At the Roots of Melancholy', 242.

the history of Western medical thought to its core psychology. Without the core psychology, it is hard to see how melancholia would have survived.

4   Melancholia from antiquity to the Renaissance

From its earliest history melancholia was part of medical theory and practice, and it was the institution of medicine that sustained it. The term *melancholia* first appears in the corpus of medical writings attributed to Hippocrates and his school. Although cognates of *melancholia* also appear in some non-medical texts of the period (notably those of the comic playwright Aristophanes, but also those of Plato and Aristotle),[10] it was almost entirely through medical texts and practices that knowledge about the disease was transmitted to later antiquity. In fact the very origin of the word was dependent on medicine. Its etymology indicates that it is a secondary and composite concept. The word *melancholia* is composed from *melainē* (black) and *cholē* (bile). In all likelihood it derives from a pre-existing medical usage of the term *cholē*. This term designates the fluid bile (or gall) which is produced by the liver and is one of a number of fluids or 'humours' that were considered important by the Greeks and may have been of even earlier ancient Near Eastern origin. (The number of these humours is usually put at four, but Hippocrates certainly knew of many more than this,[11] and the agreement on four humours was probably the result of later simplification and schematization.) For at least 200 years before the first extant use of *melancholia* by Hippocrates, the word *cholē* also had a psychological usage in the sense of *anger*, chiefly in poetry. Presumably the emotion was named *cholē* on the analogy of the unpleasant circumstances of bile rising to the throat.

Thus the early history of melancholia already presents a tension that runs through the whole tradition. As far as its etymology is concerned, *melancholia* sprang from a Greek way of thinking that accorded great medical significance to the humours. But the humours were not in themselves pathological. Indeed, properly regulated and balanced humours were a guarantee of good health. On the other hand, in the earliest Hippocratic texts, melancholia appears already to have become established as a disease in its own right, as in the following passage from one of the earliest extant writings, *Airs, Waters, Places*:

---

[10] Jouanna, 'At the Roots of Melancholy', 232–3.

[11] Claus Vogel, 'Zur Entstehung der hippokratischen *Viersäftelehre*', unpublished dissertation (Marburg, 1956), 9.

But if the weather be northerly and dry, with no rain either during the Dog Star or at Arcturus, it is very beneficial to those that have a phlegmatic or humid constitution, and to women, but it is very harmful to the bilious. For these dry up overmuch, and are attacked by dry ophthalmia and by acute, protracted fevers, in some cases too by melancholias [*melancholiai*].[12]

There is evidence here of systematic thinking about the humoral constitution of human bodies and how this constitution interacts with the climate and environment. Dry weather suits those whose constitution is naturally damp or 'phlegmatic', phlegm being a naturally watery humour. Dryness counteracts that dampness and brings the phlegmatic body's humoral constitution back into a healthy balance. Indeed, the underlying principle of most Hippocratic therapy is the application of a regimen, most often but not always dietary, that aims to restore to the body a healthy balance or mix (*krasis*).

So far, *Airs, Waters, Places* confirms the traditional view of Hippocratic medicine as rationalistic, systematic, and schematic. On the other hand, there is no evidence in *Airs, Waters, Places* of four types of constitution corresponding to the four humours (phlegm, yellow bile, blood, and black bile). There is no mention of a melancholy bodily constitution, let alone a melancholy temperament. All we find is a disease (or diseases) called melancholia. Since a substance by the name of 'black bile' is not mentioned, only diseases or cases of *melancholia*, it is reasonable to suppose that melancholia is caused not by a preponderance of black bile, as later medical writers would argue, but by normal yellow bile that has somehow turned black.[13]

According to one easy and misleading commonplace about Graeco-Roman medicine, melancholia owes its existence to a stable and universally accepted theory of the four humours. Modern medicine has shown that the theory of the four humours is untrue. Bile, phlegm, and blood do, of course, exist, but they are not connected in the ways that Graeco-Roman humoral theory says they are. Nor are they, whether individually or in combination, responsible for regulating health in the ways that Graeco-Roman physicians assumed. If the humoral theory has no basis in reality, and if melancholia owed its existence to and had always been part of the humoral theory, we would have strong grounds for an antirealist view of melancholia. But there are two reasons to reject the argument that melancholia is dependent on the humoral theory. First, as we have already seen, the disease melancholia in *Airs, Waters, Places* predates the theory of the humours. And second, the classic tetradic humoral theory was by no means fixed at the time the earliest Hippocratic texts were composed. In fact, within the Hippocratic corpus

---

[12] Hippocrates, *Airs, Waters, Places*, x, in *Hippocrates I*, 103.
[13] Flashar, *Melancholie*, 22–7; Jouanna, 'At the Roots of Melancholy', 232–3.

there were diverse opinions as to the underlying physiological and physical framework within which melancholia was to be understood. Bodies, we hear, are variously composed of two, three, or four humours; the physical world may be made of one, two, or four elements.[14] One explanation for this apparent theoretical eclecticism is that the Hippocratic physicians were guided by empirical observation to a greater extent than a later, more rationalist age was prepared to admit or give them credit for.[15] For various reasons later medical writers would schematize Hippocratic practice into the simpler tetradic model. It is highly significant therefore that, in *Airs, Waters, Places* at any rate, melancholia is a distinct, observable disease with a specific aetiology. The idea of *melancholia* derives partly from a habit of thinking about the relation of the body to its environment, and partly from empirical observation.

Only in the later writings of the Hippocratic corpus does melancholia emerge as a constitutional type (though not yet as a temperament).[16] And only in these later writings, in particular *On the Nature of Man*, which seems to have been written around 400 BC, a generation or so later than *Airs, Waters, Places*, is there evidence of an attempt to construct a systematic physiology based on the humoral fluids. Here for the first time we encounter the idea that humans consist of a mixture of four humours, which implies in turn that black bile is present not just in cases of melancholic disease, but also in healthy humans.[17] In the later books of the Hippocratic *Epidemics*, a collection of observations of cases, this melancholic type is said to suffer from a range of psychological symptoms.

The tension between these two tendencies, the systematic and the empirical, runs right through Graeco-Roman medicine. By Roman times the tendencies had polarized into two broad camps. On one side stood the *empirikoi*, who thought that the foundation of medical knowledge was whatever had been shown to work in the past, whether derived from autopsy or from critical evaluation of other physicians' reports. On the other side stood the *logikoi*. They insisted on a theoretical understanding of how and why people became ill, which in turn necessitated a theory of human physiology. These rationalist approaches used ambitious explanatory systems based on speculative reasoning, in which the functions of the body were embedded in a larger system of natural philosophy,

---

[14] Erich Schöner, *Das Viererschema in der antiken Humoralpathologie*. Südhoffs Archiv Beiheft 4 (Wiesbaden: Steiner, 1964), 57.

[15] *Ibid.*, 102.

[16] Flashar, *Melancholie*, 32–3. See also Jouanna, 'At the Roots of Melancholy', 229–36.

[17] Flashar, *Melancholie*, 39, 43.

with man at its centre.[18] Even in Hippocratic medicine there is evidence of the influence of natural philosophy, such as Empedocles' (*c.* 490–430 BC) doctrine of the four elements (fire, air, earth, and water), though, as we have seen, a range of such theories was entertained and the four-element theory was by no means an inevitable choice. Indeed, Empedocles is criticized in the Hippocratic treatise *On Ancient Medicine* precisely for importing philosophical models into medicine.[19] The Hippocratic physicians were evidently aware of the need to retain a degree of empiricism. Still, the tendency to think about medicine in terms of natural philosophy had important and long-lasting consequences. The status of natural philosophy was such that few medical writers in the Graeco-Roman rationalist tradition avoided it.

Towards the end of the classical period of Ancient Greece, melancholia became the subject of philosophical interest. Theophrastus (*c.* 371–*c.* 287 BC), who succeeded Aristotle as leader of the Peripatetic school of philosophy, is said to have written the first book entirely devoted to melancholia. There followed a hiatus during the Hellenistic period, when attention seems to have moved away from the Hippocratic humoral system, and the two prevailing philosophical schools, Epicureanism and Stoicism, were not well disposed towards melancholic psychology (as we will see in Chapter 4). Interest picked up again in the Roman era. There is evidence of extensive commentary on melancholia by the medical writers Celsus (*c.* 25-*c.* 50 BC), Aretaeus (*fl.* first century AD), Soranus (*fl.* first–second century AD), and above all Rufus of Ephesus (*fl.* late first century AD), the author of an important lost treatise *On Melancholia* in two books. (Much of the content of Rufus' *On Melancholia* can be reconstructed from passages quoted or paraphrased in later Graeco-Roman medical writers and in the authors of medical writings in Arabic.)[20] Rufus' account of melancholia appears to have influenced Galen (AD 129–199/217), the most celebrated physician of the Roman era, second in fame only to Hippocrates in antiquity, and the most prolific medical writer of antiquity.

Melancholia was not foremost among Galen's interests. His most extensive discussion of it, in Book III of *On the Affected Parts*, approaches diseases from the perspective of anatomy: it is concerned less with disease itself than with the pathophysiology of the anatomical locations of diseases. Despite his relative lack of interest in melancholia, Galen was

---

[18] Rebecca Flemming, *Medicine and the Making of Roman Women: Gender, Nature and Authority from Celsus to Galen* (Oxford University Press, 2000), 89.

[19] Schöner, *Viererschema*, 4–13.

[20] See the edition in Rufus of Ephesus, *On Melancholy*, ed. Peter E. Pormann, SAPERE XII (Tübingen: Mohr Siebeck, 2008).

responsible for one of the most significant moves towards its schematization – namely, the assumption that there are four psychological types
corresponding to the four humours. Thus the black bile is associated
with a melancholy character type that is 'steady and constant'. (This is
very different from most later versions of the melancholy character: for
instance, Vindicianus, *fl.* AD 400, characterized melancholics as fearful
and sad.)[21] The mapping of four character types onto the four humours
was itself part of a more general process of schematization, whereby a
series of tetrads from different realms of nature were mapped onto one
another. Galen linked the four humours to four skin colours, four organs,
and four ages of man, although it should be said that he did on occasion
express reservations about some of these correspondences.[22] The process
of schematization continued with the sixth-century *On the Humours* (erroneously attributed to Galen) and the anonymous *On the Nature of the
Universe [and] Man.* Here the humours and character types became linked
to the four elements (earth is the element corresponding to melancholia),
the four qualities (hot, dry, cold, and wet: melancholia partakes of both
the cold and the dry), and the four seasons (melancholia is linked to
autumn: contrast Hippocrates' argument in *Airs, Waters, Places* that melancholia affects bilious people in the summer). Eventually pretty much
anything that could be formed into a group of four would be added to the
scheme: astrological signs (second century AD) and points of the compass
(seventh century AD).[23] From the ninth century dates the tradition of
linking melancholia with the god Saturn.[24]

In Galenism, melancholia became something more than just a disease
or even a physiological substance. It became a character type, a temperament, and as such it had potential applications in other discourses beyond
medicine, notably in ethics and poetry. The end result of this process of
diffusion is the English usage of the term *melancholy* we discussed above,
in which determinate clinical content has been all but swamped by
broader cultural usages. In one sense this can be read as a sign of the
power of melancholia – its capacity to extend its uses far beyond medicine.
But it was also a potential weakness, as it resulted in a loss of focus. A term
whose uses have become as widely diffused as has those of *melancholia* will
eventually lose its conceptual centre.[25] Diffusion can cause diffuseness.
The process of diffusion creates a vacuum at the heart of the concept
which another term can fill. In this case the other term was *depression,*

[21] Flashar, *Melancholie*, 109.   [22] Schöner, *Viererschema*, 92–3.   [23] *Ibid.*, 97–9.
[24] Flashar, *Melancholie*, 136.
[25] Siegfried Wenzel, *The Sin of Sloth: Acedia in Medieval Thought and Literature* (Chapel Hill, NC: University of North Carolina Press, 1967), 186.

which had the virtue of having a manifestly clear conceptual centre, represented not least by its strikingly expressive name. This is all part of the ebb and flow of conceptual traditions. Arguably, diffuseness is one of the problems facing *depression* now. It is being asked to do too much work over too broad a range, and its conceptual focus has become blurred.

Late antiquity saw the triumph of the Galenic system, not, it should be said, Galen's actual practice, but a simplified and still further systematized Galenism. Why did Galenism triumph? The fourth-century physician Oribasius (*c.* AD 320–400), himself the author of a collection of excerpts from Galen's writings and those of other earlier medical writers, held Galen to be supreme 'because he use[d] the most accurate methods and definitions by following the Hippocratic principles and opinions'.[26] Galen believed in the cumulative progress of medical science, but progress could proceed, he thought, only out of principles rooted in the wisdom of the ancients, above all Hippocrates.[27] The incontestable authority of Hippocrates provided a firm theoretical foundation, on which Galen could build his massive systematic edifice. But the Hippocratic writings also required interpretation, and Galen positioned himself as the sole heir and interpreter of Hippocrates, a position later medicine would largely accept, so that Galen's commentaries on Hippocrates themselves became part of the Hippocratic canon.[28]

Galenic medicine could also claim to be philosophical and systematic, and this systematic ambition enhanced its reputation. If many later physicians could not accept Galen's natural philosophy – medieval Arab and European medical writers preferred Aristotle's philosophy of nature to Galen's – at least Galenism *was* philosophical. This preference for philosophical systematicity had taken root during the Hellenistic and Roman periods. Aristotle had posited a systematic connection of the four qualities (hot, wet, cold, and dry) with the four elements (fire, water, earth, and air), and of the four qualities with the two genders (men were hot and dry, women cold and wet).[29] Physiological theorizing of this kind strengthened the link between medical practice and philosophy. The physicians also had institutional reasons for drawing on natural philosophy. Theory enhanced medicine's aura of professionalism. An important reason for the triumph of Galenism was its theoretical structure, the parading of which made the physician seem clearly superior to the quack and so gave confidence to his patients.[30] Untheoretical medical schools, such as the *empirikoi* and the methodists, who rejected aetiology and experiment and

[26] Owsei Temkin, *Galenism: Rise and Decline of a Medical Philosophy* (Ithaca, NY: Cornell University Press, 1973), 62.
[27] *Ibid.*, 31.   [28] *Ibid.*, 32.   [29] Schöner, *Viererschema*, 20.   [30] Temkin, *Galenism*, 124.

inferred directly from symptoms to the state of a patient's health, could be derided as reckless amateurs.[31] Virtuous theory supported Galen's attacks on unprofessional contemporary physicians' greed, lust for power, and so on.[32] Being (or seeming to be) philosophical conferred a competitive advantage, regardless whether it actually helped to cure patients. This also lies at the root of the traditional distinction between the profession of the physician and that of the surgeon, and the higher status of the former. The distinction lasted into the eighteenth century. The physician offered opinions grounded in theory, often from the comfortable distance of his study and in the form of a letter for which he might charge a substantial sum. Sir Hans Sloane charged a guinea a letter.[33] The surgeon was of lower status, a craftsman who practised the messier business of fixing broken limbs and dressing wounds.

At the end of antiquity medicine was effectively united under Galen's name. This was the tradition that survived in the Greek-speaking Eastern Roman Empire, while the Latin-speaking Western Empire fell into the Dark Ages and lost contact with the East. In the intellectual centres of the Eastern Empire, principally Constantinople and Alexandria, Galenism lived on, digested and recompiled by physicians such as Oribasius, Alexander of Tralles (c. AD 525–c. 605), Aëtius of Amida (fl. mid-fifth to mid-sixth century AD), and Paul of Aegina (c. AD 625–c. 690). From the Eastern Empire, Galenism spread into the Islamic Middle East, whence it would eventually return to Western Europe via the Islamic Maghreb, Spain, Sicily, and southern Italy in the eleventh century AD. In the Middle East, Galenism was transmitted via Byzantine compilations of Galen,[34] which were then translated first into Syriac, then Arabic. The *Isagoge* of Ḥunain ibn Isḥāq (Johannitius, 809–873), the first translator of Greek medicine into Arabic, was a highly simplified and schematized introduction to Galen based on Alexandrian synopses of Galen's writings.[35] The first significant work of Western European medicine on melancholia, written by Constantinus Africanus (1017–1087) at the southern Italian medical school of Salerno, was in fact a translation of Isḥāq ibn 'Imrān's *On Melancholia* (*Maqāla fī'l-mālīḫūliyā*),[36] which was in turn heavily dependent on (and is one of the chief sources for reconstructing) Rufus' *On Melancholia*.[37]

---

[31] *Ibid.*, 31–2.   [32] *Ibid.*, 35–6.

[33] See, for instance, William Dobson to Sir Hans Sloane, 12 September 1730, London, British Library, MS Sloane 4075, fol. 79.

[34] Jackson, *Melancholia and Depression*, 48.   [35] Temkin, *Galenism*, 106.

[36] Karl Garbers, 'Einleitung', in Isḥāq ibn 'Imrān, *Maqāla fī'l-mālīḫūliyā*, xiii–xxxvii (at pp. xxxii–xxxiii).

[37] Peter E. Pormann, 'Introduction', in Rufus of Ephesus, *On Melancholy*, 3–23 (at p. 14).

By the early Middle Ages the tradition of melancholia in Western Europe hung by a slender thread. What knowledge of melancholia there was, principally Constantinus Africanus' *On Melancholia*, derived from repeatedly translated and summarized versions of long-lost Greek originals. The Arab physicians had made some contributions to the tradition. In particular they extended the range of herbal and chemical treatments available to the physician, the so-called *materia medica*. But the theory appears to have ossified. The slender basis of the tradition in the medieval West was further attenuated by another factor, the lack of knowledge of the Ancient Greek language, not that the Greek texts were available to read in any case. But knowledge of Greek would at least have given medieval physicians a sense of where *melancholia* came from. Ignorance of the Greek language meant that the origins of the tradition, inscribed in the etymological sense of *melancholia* as black bile, became utterly obscure. There was therefore nothing to prevent the medieval vernacular European languages in which *melancholia* first gained a foothold, notably Italian and French, from thoroughly assimilating the word to their own linguistic morphology and so obscuring its original meaning even further. Medieval Italian produced *malinconia* and even *maninconia*. Medieval French had *mérencolye*. *Melancholia* was not the only victim of this process of linguistic oblivion, and other elements of Greek psychiatry suffered a similar fate. The term *phrenitis*, denoting a feverish disease of the brain leading to madness, from the Greek noun *phrēn* (brain), was transliterated into Arabic as *farānītis*, whence it mutated into *qarānītis*. When the *Canon of Medicine* of Avicenna (Ibn Sīnā, *c.* 980–1037) was translated into Latin, *qarānītis* became the mysterious disease of *karabitus*.[38] This was a linguistically disinherited tradition.

The Western Middle Ages canonized a single, debased version of the melancholy tradition, essentially a Galenized version of Rufus of Ephesus, transmitted via Byzantine compilations that were then translated into Arabic and Latin. In the process the polyphony of Graeco-Roman medicine was replaced by near unanimity. Medicine was heavily systematized and brought into line with Aristotelian natural philosophy and astrology. This systematic edifice was then projected back onto Hippocrates. The effect was to suggest that there was and always had been only one medical truth, and that this truth had the sanction of antiquity. (Even some modern historians of melancholia have claimed that the fully worked out tetradic humoral scheme, if not explicitly mentioned by Hippocrates, is at least there by implication.)[39] Why the obsession with unanimity? In the

---

[38] Manfred Ullmann, *Islamic Medicine* (Edinburgh University Press, 1978), 29.
[39] See, for instance, Klibansky, Panofsky, and Saxl, *Saturn and Melancholy*, 4–13.

first place, it was a natural effect of the medium in which much medical knowledge was transmitted – namely, summaries and excerpts from earlier writers. The process of excerpting led to homogenization, for the excerpters were never scrupulous about indicating their sources (why should they be?) and so revealing the actual diversity of ancient opinions. The process was assisted by the passage of time, and in particular the fall of the Roman Empire. Historical and cultural distance caused the past to lose its contours. Once the melancholy tradition had passed out of Graeco-Roman antiquity and into the Islamo-Christian era, some simplification was inevitable. From this distance antiquity increasingly looked like one homogeneous thing and ancient medicine one coherent and consistent body of thought. This resulted in the assumption that the ancient medical writers had in fact all believed essentially the same thing. The job of the excerpter or compiler of medical texts was therefore to find this single truth and to deny or explain away any apparent disagreements between the sources. The work of 'reconciling the sources' became a significant industry in late medieval and early modern Europe. No doubt the relatively monolithic nature of the monotheistic medieval West, at least in contrast to the regionally highly varied religious and cultural life of polytheistic Ancient Greece and Rome, played some part in this. Just as now there was (in theory) a single Catholic theological and a single neo-Aristotelian philosophical truth, so there must be a single Galenic medical truth. The Renaissance and Reformation may have diluted this effect somewhat by insisting on a return to what Hippocrates and Galen actually wrote, and thus revealing once again the polyphony of ancient medicine, but the schism of the Reformation was to generate its own neuroses about the fragmentation of culture and provoke a countervailing drive to reinstate the one true wisdom.[40]

The effect on melancholia of the Renaissance and Reformation was twofold. The drive to restore pristine ancient knowledge had profound effects on medicine. In his *Invective Against the Doctor*, Petrarch (1304–1374) attacked modern physicians for abandoning medicine's 'ancient glory'.[41] Niccolò Leoniceno (1428–1524) voiced scepticism about modern medical terminology and argued for a return to the purity of the sources.[42] The great Dutch humanist Erasmus sponsored the five-volume Aldine edition of Galen (1525), including in volume IV the first attempt at

[40] Angus Gowland, *The Worlds of Renaissance Melancholy: Robert Burton in Context* (New York: Cambridge University Press, 2006), 29–34.
[41] Cited in Gowland, *Worlds*, 101.
[42] Roy Porter, *The Greatest Benefit to Mankind: A Medical History of Humanity from Antiquity to the Present* (London: HarperCollins, 1997), 170–1.

a systematic list of works once attributed to Galen but now deemed spurious, a significant departure.[43] The return to sources could reveal diversity rather than the hoped-for pure Galenic unanimity. Although Galenism remained dominant – during the sixteenth century, 590 printings of Galen are known to have been produced in Western Europe – Hippocrates was also now being published independently in Latin (from 1525) and Greek (from 1526), providing competition for Galen and raising the possibility that disagreements between the two great medical authorities might come to light,[44] although even in the seventeenth century much energy was still being devoted to proving that all classical physicians believed essentially the same thing, so strong was the magisterial authority of antiquity.

The newly apparent diversity of opinion among the ancients had another unintended effect: to create space for new modern theories. If the ancient authorities could not agree, why should the moderns feel bound to do so? The first significant challenges to the ancient medical tradition arose in the sixteenth century, notably the chemical-based theory of Paracelsus (Philippus Aureolus Theophrastus Bombastus von Hohenheim, 1493–1541).[45] But the most significant change came with the rediscovery by the Florentine Neoplatonist philosopher Marsilio Ficino (1433–1499) of a Greek text on melancholia probably by Theophrastus (though until recently it was attributed to Aristotle). This text, *Problems* XXX/1, which had been almost entirely ignored in antiquity, presented a theory that would revolutionize the nature and status of melancholia in early modern Europe. By linking melancholia to creative genius, it opened a vast new field of potential cultural applications, and at the same time precipitated melancholia's slide into conceptual diffuseness.

5   *Depression* from antiquity to 1900

The history of the word *depression* was entirely unlike and largely separate from that of *melancholia*, at least for its first 2,000 years. *Melancholia* was a medical term that spawned non-medical uses. *Depression* was a non-medical term that gradually infiltrated medicine by virtue of its metaphorical force. From antiquity to the early modern period, *depression* had a long linguistic history, before it became a medical concept in the eighteenth and nineteenth centuries. This pre-medical usage of *depression* belonged to everyday folk psychological language. Its nature was originally

---

[43] *Ibid.*, 169.   [44] *Ibid.*, 171.   [45] Temkin, *Galenism*, 128–9.

metaphorical. It was one of a group of related metaphorical usages, some of which were connected to *melancholia*, while others were not. Even in the nineteenth century, when the theory of the black bile had finally been superseded, depression was still subordinate to melancholia in the hierarchy of psychiatric nosology. It was only around 1900 that depression began to replace melancholia as a top-level nosological category.

It could be argued that *melancholia* also contains a metaphorical element – namely, 'black' (*melas, melainē*), which is in turn connected to a whole range of psychological metaphors of darkness (gloom, the black dog, the blues, and so on). However, these were in most cases secondary to and consequent on the medical theory of the black bile. Thus, when in antiquity it was claimed that a dark view of the world was characteristic of melancholia, this was held to be because the black vapours produced by burnt bile clouded the sight or brain. (The rationality and usefulness of these metaphors was much discussed in the early modern medical literature.)[46] Unlike *melancholia, depression* originated outside medical discourse. And it originated quite independently at different times and in different places. Its multiple independent origins and the way it insinuated itself into medicine are evidence of its exceptional power (though, as we will see, its climb to the top of the nosological hierarchy was by no means inevitable). *Depression* and related metaphors would appear to belong to a species of metaphors that naturally force themselves on us. To be sure, there was also an element of traditional usage in these metaphors, which was dictated by literary traditions or common cultural norms. In other words, people used *depression* as a metaphor because it was felt to have creative potential, but also because it was part of traditional literary language. Still, the natural vigour of the metaphor *depression* is demonstrated by the fact that this traditional usage, once established, was able to sustain itself until the nineteenth century without any institutional support from medicine.

In their folk psychological senses *depression* and its cognates contain two metaphors: downward motion or orientation (*de-*) and pressure, weight, and mass (*press-*). The use of metaphors of weight to describe mental unease is of great antiquity. In a fragment of a lost post-Homeric epic on the sack of Troy, reputedly by Arctinus of Miletus (perhaps *fl. c.* 750 BC), the mad Ajax is described as having a 'mind weighed down' (*barunomenon noēma*).[47] Similar metaphors of weight and pressure are attested in

---

[46] Michael Kutzer, *Anatomie des Wahnsinns: Geisteskrankheit im medizinischen Denken der frühen Neuzeit und die Anfänge der pathologischen Anatomie* (Hürtgenwald: Pressler, 1998), 115–17, 119.

[47] *Sack of Ilion*, fragment 2, line 8, in *Greek Epic Fragments*, ed. and trans. M. L. West, Loeb Classical Library (Cambridge, MA: Harvard University Press, 2003), 149.

Latin.[48] The Latin ancestor of the English word 'depressed', *depressus*, was used in this sense, with the connotation of having been overcome by a dominant and inimical force.[49] In medieval and modern times the folk psychological metaphor of heaviness is most obvious in German. The word *Schwermut* (literally 'heavy-spiritedness'), denoting grief, depression, and related states, is attested as early as the thirteenth century and has been in common use ever since. In the early modern period, *Schwermut* was used as a synonym of *Melancholie*: in Zedler's 66-volume *Universal Lexicon* of the mid eighteenth century, the article 'Schwermut' refers the reader to the article 'Melancholie'.[50] However, *Schwermut* never established itself as a formal nosological category.

Metaphors of downward motion or orientation are as ancient as those of weight and pressure. The adjective *katēphēs* meaning 'downcast' appears in the *Odyssey*.[51] The prefix *kat-* here denotes 'down'. Originally the word appears to have referred specifically to the downwards cast of the eyes. The second element, *-phēs*, apparently derives from *phaos*, 'light' or 'eyes' when in the plural. Indeed, downcast eyes have an even longer history. Even in the ancient Near Eastern Gilgamesh epics, downcast eyes are connected with grief. Mourning the death of his dear friend Enkidu, Gilgamesh roams the open countryside in tattered clothes and is quizzed on his bizarre behaviour:

> Ur-shanabi spoke to him, to Gilgamesh,
> 'Why are your cheeks wasted, your face dejected,
> Your heart so wretched, your appearance worn out,
> And grief in your innermost being?'[52]

The Akkadian word *quddudu*, translated here as 'dejected', derives from a verb meaning 'to bow, to bend down, to incline'.[53]

In other words, the association of profound sadness with downward orientation of the eyes or face must have originated independently on multiple occasions. It was a natural metaphor. It also became part of the classical tradition. The Latin absolute phrase 'with eyes cast down to the ground' (*demissis* [also *deiectis*] *in terram oculis*) seems to have become a set

---

[48] For example, Curtius, *Historia Alexandri Magni*, 4, 13, 17; Cicero, *Pro Cluentio*, 58.
[49] Cicero, *De senectute*, 77.
[50] Johann Heinrich Zedler, *Grosses vollständiges Universal-Lexicon aller Wissenschafften und Künste, welche bishero durch menschlichen Verstand und Witz erfunden und verbessert worden*, 66 vols. (Leipzig and Halle: Zedler, 1732–52), vol. XXXVI, coll. 464–76.
[51] Homer, *Odyssey*, XXIV, 432; also Euripides, *Herakles*, 633.
[52] Stephanie Dalley (ed.), *Myths from Mesopotamia: Creation, The Flood, Gilgamesh, and Others* (Oxford University Press, 1989), 103.
[53] I am most grateful to Dr Stephanie Dalley for her help with the Akkadian meaning of this passage.

phrase.[54] It had two meanings, which were probably not distinguished at first. Downcast eyes can signify both dejection and shame (or modesty). Later these would separate into two distinct usages, with the 'shame' meaning relating in particular to female modesty.[55] Downcast eyes would become part of the stock iconography of melancholia. Rufus uses the adjective *katēphēs* to describe the melancholic.[56] Much later, downcast eyes appear repeatedly in the Renaissance, whether in Dürer's etching *Melencolia I* or Shakespeare's plays. The motif of downcast eyes was also connected with another stock element of melancholy iconography, the dark face. The connection may have arisen because the face was downcast and thus in shadow or because the face got a livid hue from black bile.

The term *depression*, deriving by analogy from the twin metaphorical traditions of 'down' and 'weighed', would eventually enter into medical usage. Its earliest medical use in English is in the stock phrase 'depression of spirits', which is frequently attested from the seventeenth century onwards. Often depression of spirits was associated with a mental disorder, whether as a symptom of melancholia, hypochondria, or insanity,[57] or as one of a cluster of symptoms including melancholia, hypochondria, or anxiety. Still, depression of spirits had no nosological standing. Unlike melancholia and hypochondria, but in common with anxiety, depression was not considered a disease in its own right. And the diseases of which it was a symptom, such as smallpox or scarlet fever, might be quite unrelated to mental illness.[58] Or depression of spirits might be the result of some influence that affected the constitution as a whole, such as tea drinking or hot or cold bathing.[59] In this sense, depression of spirits was a transient though potentially long-lasting state, but not a permanent one. You could experience a bout of depression of spirits, perhaps lasting for years, but you could not be constitutionally depressed of spirits. This is because *depression* denoted an interruption in normal physiological functioning, such as an episode of lassitude or a reduction in the strength or activity of the 'animal spirits'.[60] However, depression of spirits could be the result of

---

[54] Seneca the Elder, *Controversiae*, 2, 4, 3; Tacitus, *Annales*, 1, 34, 1, and *Historiae*, 3, 31, 3.

[55] Curtius, *Historia Alexandri Magni*, 6, 2, 6.   [56] Klibansky *et al.*, *Saturn*, 50.

[57] William Perfect, *Cases of Insanity, The Epilepsy, Hypochondriacal Affection, Hysteric Passion, and Nervous Disorders, Successfully Treated* (Rochester: Fisher, 1785), 7, 163, and *Select Cases in the Different Species of Insanity, Lunacy, or Madness, with the Modes of Practice as Adopted in the Treatment of Each* (Rochester: Gillman, 1787), 169, 259, 311.

[58] John Gregory, *Elements of the Practice of Physic* (Edinburgh: Balfour and Smellie, 1788), 51, 62, 88, 112, 114.

[59] Tea drinking: Anon., *An Essay on the Nature, Use, and Abuse, of Tea, in a Letter to a Lady; With an Account of its Mechanical Operation* (London: Bettenham, 1722), 32. Bathing: John King, *An Essay on Hot and Cold Bathing* (London: Bettenham, 1737), 111.

[60] George Cheyne, *An Essay of Health and Long Life* (Dublin: Wilmot, 1725), 100.

a physical or psychological state. In the latter case, a transient depression of spirits might be caused by excessive passions, religious enthusiasm, or superstition.[61] By the late eighteenth century this latter type of depression had acquired a wide usage well beyond technical medical writings: depression of spirits appears in religious sermons, biographies and memoirs, and novels.[62]

The rise of depression in the eighteenth and nineteenth centuries was due in the first place to its own metaphorical force, but a shift in medical physiology away from traditional humoral theory opened cracks into which depression could seep. The theory of the four humours was first seriously undermined by the conclusive demonstration of the circulation of the blood by William Harvey in the early seventeenth century. It was now clear that blood was far more significant for the general constitution than the other humours were. But it was the growing focus on the nerves and their functions, beginning in the late seventeenth century, that fatally undermined traditional humoral theory. Rather than an imbalance of the humours, disease was now understood in terms of an excess or deficit of nervous tension. The last quarter of the eighteenth century saw a rise in the diagnosis of asthenia, a weakness or under-stimulation of the nerves. In this context depression became increasingly common as a symptom: it occupied progressively more space at the bottom of the nosological pyramid, as it were. The rise of depression was very much a *rise* – from the bottom up.

What of the categories at the top of the pyramid? In antiquity mental disorders were normally divided into three categories, one feverish

---

[61] Excessive passions: Samuel Johnson, *A Dictionary of the English Language: In which the Words are Deduced from their Originals, and Illustrated in their Different Significations, by Examples from the Best Writers, to which are Prefixed a History of the Language, and an English Grammar*, 2 vols. (London: Strahan, 1755–6), vol. I, unpaginated, article 'depress'. Enthusiasm: Thomas Green, *A Dissertation on Enthusiasm; Shewing the Danger of its Late Increase, and the Great Mischiefs it has Occasioned, both in Ancient and Modern Times* (London: Oliver, 1755), 114. Superstition: David Hume, 'Of Superstition and Enthusiasm', in Hume, *Essays Moral, Political, and Literary*, 4 vols. (London: Millar, 1760), vol. I, 127.

[62] Sermons: Thomas Harmer, *The Good Liable to Intellectual Disorders, of the Melancholy Kind, Equally with Others: A Sermon* (London: Hawes, 1779), 14, 17. Memoirs: J. Langhorne, 'Memoirs of the Author', in *The Poetical Works of Mr William Collins. With Memoirs of the Author; and Observations on his Genius and Writings* (London: Becket, 1771), xiii. The term occurs with predictable frequency in the novels of Charlotte Smith: *Emmeline; Or the Orphan of the Castle* (London: Cadell, 1788), vol. III, 116; *Etheline; Or the Recluse of the Lake* (London: Cadell, 1789), vol. I, 200; *Celestina*, 2nd edn (London: Cadell, 1791), vol. IV, 212; *Desmond* (London: Robinson, 1792), vol. II, 17; *The Old Manor House* (London: Bell, 1793), vol. III, 99; vol. IV, 267; *The Wanderings of Warwick* (London: Bell, 1794), 33; *Montalbert* (London: Low, 1795), vol. II, 155; vol. III, 114; *Marchmont* (London: Low, 1796), vol. IV, 24.

(phrenitis) and two non-feverish (melancholia and mania). The Galenic tradition tended to uphold this tripartite division and with it the prominent position of melancholia on the non-feverish side. To be sure, there were those such as Burton who idiosyncratically lumped all mental illness together under melancholia. On the other hand, the tendency towards innovation in theory and diagnosis in the modern period, especially in the agitated atmosphere of revolutionary France, began to threaten the primacy of melancholia. In his *Traité médico-philosophique sur l'aliénation mentale; ou la manie* (1801), Philippe Pinel used four top-level categories of mental illness: mania, dementia, melancholia, and imbecility. Pinel's pupil Jean-Étienne Dominique Esquirol went further. In his 1838 *Des maladies mentales*, Esquirol proposed replacing melancholia with a new category of his own invention, 'lypemania' (from the Greek *lupē*: pain, distress, grief), but this was an innovation too far and did not catch on.

Esquirol's lypemania nicely illustrates a shift around 1800 in the status of the classical tradition in general and the Hippocratic-Galenic medical tradition in particular. The authority of the ancient physicians had long gone more or less unchallenged, even where there was no empirical evidence to support it. One of the forms of melancholia reported in antiquity was lycanthropia or the delusion that the sufferer is a wolf. In serious cases this was believed to cause wolf-like behaviour such as hanging about in graveyards at night and howling at the moon. Lycanthropia remained in medical nosologies well into the eighteenth century and beyond under the traditional category 'wandering melancholia' (*melancholia errabunda*).[63] Throughout its history lycanthropia was a very traditional disease, in the sense that reports of cases were usually recycled from the earlier sources.[64] Most medical writers who wrote about lycanthropia appear never to have seen or heard of a case of it, outside their reading of the traditional medical literature. They simply rehashed the reports they found in the ancient sources. After 1800 this began to change. Lycanthropia began to disappear from the textbooks, but the structure that had created it, the classification of zoanthropic delusions under the heading of melancholia, remained intact. By the middle of the nineteenth century hippanthropia had become the most common zoanthropic delusion. Wolves were being eradicated from Western Europe and were therefore less present to the European mind. It may be that thinking oneself a

---

[63] It was still in use in the mid nineteenth century: Heinrich August Pierer, *Universal-Lexikon der Vergangenheit und Gegenwart, oder Neuestes encyclopädisches Wörterbuch der Wissenschaften, Künste und Gewerbe*, 4th edn, 19 vols. (Altenburg: Pierer, 1857–65), in the article 'Geisteskrankheiten', vol. VII, 86.

[64] Jackson, *Melancholia*, 345–51.

horse was more in tune with modern European culture. So the classical tradition survived as a zoanthropic framework, only now filled with modern contents. The authority of Hippocrates and Galen was on the wane. Individual theories and classifications were challenged. But a belief in the enduring spirit of classical medicine persisted. Esquirol's lypemania is a case in point.

Melancholia, though challenged by Pinel, Esquirol, and others, remained the dominant category for non-feverish mental illness until end of nineteenth century. It was only in the work of Emil Kraepelin (1856–1926) that depression replaced melancholia. In the sixth edition of his *Lehrbuch der Psychiatrie* (*Textbook of Psychiatry*, 1899), Kraepelin recategorized melancholic conditions on a completely new scheme. Most were now relocated under the category of 'manic-depressive psychoses'. The category melancholia was reserved for 'involutional', that is, externally caused, melancholia. In the eighth edition (1909–13) the category melancholia was abandoned altogether.[65] Melancholia disappeared from the top level of psychiatric diagnosis. And so it has remained more or less ever since. With Kraepelin depression came to occupy positions both at the bottom *and* at the top of the diagnostic pyramid. During the hundred years since Kraepelin it has occupied virtually all the territory in between.

6   The end of melancholia

What are the key factors in the conceptual history we have outlined here? One way to read the story of melancholia and depression would be to focus on the relation between theoretical entities and metaphors. In its sense of black bile, *melancholia* was a descriptive term for a theoretical entity (though its relation to the entity it purported to describe was not without problems, as we will see in Chapter 2). Once the idea of bile's blackness had become fixed in medical discourse, it began to generate its own set of metaphors of darkness, such as the idea of a darkened perception of the world or a gloomy cast of mind. These metaphors have been hugely influential; we still live with them. This serves as a reminder that the medical tradition of humoralism, with its seemingly tenuous basis in fact, has been constantly confirmed and reinforced by folk psychological observation. Although the Galenic theory of melancholia was in some ways highly traditional and theoretical, throughout its long history it continued to receive empirical confirmation. If there is one sense in which psychiatry is different from other sciences or indeed other fields

---

[65] *Ibid.*, 188–95.

of medicine, it is that the objects of psychiatric study are constantly and directly present to us in our own and others' minds. A fairly basic form of folk psychiatric observation is constantly available to us. Meaningful empirical contributions – again, I emphasize, at a basic level – can be made without any special technical preparation.

If melancholia was a descriptive label that generated new facts metaphorically, the case of depression is rather different. Depression moved in the opposite direction. It was originally a metaphor that turned into a scientific concept. It did so by attaching itself to phenomena that were already established objects of medical study, notably the symptoms of melancholia. On the one hand, depression is a good example of the process whereby scientific theories coalesce out of metaphorical talk.[66] And on the other hand, depression owes its success to its parasitic dependence on the Graeco-Roman tradition of melancholia.

The more recent fate of the two concepts has also been very different. As *melancholia* became *melancholy*, took on broader cultural meanings, and lost its conceptual focus, it became less useful as a medical term. It ended up carrying too much non-medical, cultural baggage. One of *depression*'s advantages was that, while it had a broad base in everyday and medical usage, it did not have the kind of cultural baggage that might interfere with its medical usage. Only now that much of that cultural baggage has been shed – melancholia still has a cultural profile, but it is much less prominent now than a hundred years ago: the term *melancholy* is now rather quaint – can melancholia begin to make its way back into serious contention as a medical concept. Arguably, melancholia has had to go through a period of eclipse in order to be capable of being revived as a medical category.

In view of all this, one must be wary of overstating the inevitability of melancholia's decline. It proved a remarkably tenacious top-level nosological category, remaining in clinical use beyond 1900. Its continued high standing in psychiatric nosology was due partly to institutional sociology. It survived thanks to the long-standing primacy of theory over observation among physicians and thanks to the authority of antiquity. But after 1800 the authority of antiquity began to crumble rapidly. In particular, while antiquity as a general idea retained some prestige, the authority of the most eminent ancient medical writers, Hippocrates and Galen, weakened considerably. In the end melancholia suffered the same fate as the classical tradition.

[66] Kutzer, *Anatomie des Wahnsinns*, 120–1 and especially 127.

1   Depression: a disorder of mind or body?

Recent attempts to rehabilitate melancholia (e.g. by Taylor and Fink) have pointed to its distinctive physiological profile. 'Melancholic' patients typically suffer from depressed levels of the hormone cortisol. The underlying physiological condition generates the psychological symptoms of depression, but the physiological condition is the real root of the illness. This has implications not just for diagnosis but also for treatment. Because the physiological malaise is the real underlying disease, a successful treatment regime should take the form of physical interventions. Hippocrates had used the traditional methods of realigning the body's constitution through diet (solid and liquid), exercise, sleep, and environmental surroundings. Galen would later schematize these as the six 'non-natural' principles of hygiene – 'non-natural' in the sense that they were external to the physical constitution of the body. The six non-naturals were ambient air, food and drink, exercise, sleep, excretion, and disturbances of the psyche. These were the points at which Graeco-Roman physicians targeted their interventions.

Taylor and Fink's preferred form of intervention is electroconvulsive therapy (ECT). It is worth stressing that ECT is a highly controversial treatment. The chief controversy surrounds issues of consent and side effects. A study conducted in Scotland in 2008 indicated that 23 per cent of patients treated with ECT were not capable of giving fully informed consent.[1] This is because ECT is often used as a treatment of last resort in cases of profound mental disturbance, and profoundly disturbed patients are often unable to give informed consent. The documented side effects of ECT have included memory loss, long-term impairment of general cognition, and, in a very small number of cases, death. Because of the frequent absence of consent, the deadening side effects, and not least the

---

[1] *Scottish ECT Accreditation Network Annual Report 2009. Reporting on 2008* (Edinburgh: NHS National Services Scotland, 2009), 9 (www.sean.org.uk/SEANReport2009.pdf).

violence of the treatment itself, the treatment is felt by many to be brutalizing and dehumanizing. Fictive representations of ECT – for instance, the shock therapy given to the character played by Jack Nicholson in the film *One Flew over the Cuckoo's Nest* (1975) – have cemented this image in the public consciousness, though it should be stressed that ECT as it is currently practised is considerably more humane than it was in the 1970s. Nevertheless, like the fashion for lobotomy in the 1940s and 1950s, ECT has become a symbol of a psychiatric profession that has spun free of its socially responsible moorings and forgotten the Hippocratic injunction to do no harm.

Taylor and Fink's preference for ECT offers one example of how the contemporary epidemic of depression has forced scientists, health professionals, and governments to rethink their approach to treatment, and in some cases embrace unfashionable solutions. While Taylor and Fink advocate ECT and are sceptical about psychotherapy in treating severe melancholia, the UK government's National Institute of Health and Clinical Excellence (NICE) recommends that patients with moderate or severe depression should be given a blend of antidepressants and therapy.[2] Taylor and Fink are clear that melancholia is at root a physiological illness, but NICE seems to equivocate between the physical and psychological. A sceptic might conclude that NICE's approach is scattergun: it makes sense to hit depression from all sides, using all the weapons at our disposal, because we do not really know what depression is. It is like those scenes in science-fiction films: faced with a new species of hostile alien, the humans let fly with their entire arsenal of weapons until they find one that works, usually by chance. Depression is one of these aliens: mysterious, terrifying, resistant to conventional weaponry. Part of the mystery of depression is its dual nature, both physical and mental. We do not really know how ECT acts on psychological symptoms, any more than we know how antidepressants work (assuming they work at all), despite the seemingly precise model of selective serotonin reuptake inhibition promulgated by the pharmaceutical companies.[3] And even if the molecular physiology of brain states caused by ECT or SSRIs could be shown to be consistent with behavioural changes in patients, we would still be none the wiser about the connection between brain chemistry on the one hand and mood and cognitive states on the other. Our ignorance about the relation

---

[2] *Depression: Treatment and Management of Depression in Adults, Including Adults with a Chronic Physical Health Problem*, CG90 and 91 (London: National Institute for Health and Clinical Excellence, 2009), 5.
[3] See, for example, David Healy, *The Antidepressant Era* (Cambridge, MA: Harvard University Press, 1997), and Irving Kirsch, *The Emperor's New Drugs: Exploding the Antidepressant Myth* (London: The Bodley Head, 2009).

of the mind to the body is at the core of the problem of depression: the expert consensus is that depression causes changes in both brain physiology and behaviour. But where precisely is the seat of the illness?

2   The elusiveness of melancholia

Traditional melancholia is no less elusive. An ambivalence between psychological and physiological explanations can be found throughout the tradition. Often it is not only unclear what melancholia is supposed to be; it is unclear whether it exists at all. Its long history offers plenty of indications that melancholia is not a real disease, and that in any given period of history it might instead be an artefact of whatever medical theories happened to be in vogue. On the other hand, we have seen evidence of a remarkable consistency in the psychological symptoms. Some of this consistency might be the result of the authority of tradition, but some – as we saw in the case of the downcast eye – is surely due to empirical regularities. In this sense melancholia possesses its own duality: it is both a traditional body of theory grounded in the authority of Graeco-Roman medicine but responsive to new fashions in physiological science, *and* an empirical science that constantly renews itself with reference to a stable perceived reality. At the risk of being overly schematic, one might say that this duality of the traditional and the empirical corresponds roughly to the duality of mind and body. The physical theories are either largely traditional in nature (e.g. the humours) or are generated by trends in physiological science (e.g. the serotonin theory). By contrast, the psychological symptoms (e.g. the downcast eye) derive from observation. As we will see in the following sections, the correspondence is by no means complete or exact. Sometimes the converse is the case. The history of melancholia throws up physiological theories that are grounded in empirical observation as well as psychological theories that lack any empirical warrant. But more often than not we find that the psychological models make more plausible claims to empirical warrant than the physiological models do. And in light of the realism about mental disorders that I sketched in the Introduction, this makes good sense. We would expect to find more consistency and reliability in the psychological models of melancholia than in the 'parade' of physiological theories.

The traditional humoral physiology of the black bile sounds reassuringly solid but is in fact elusive. It is questionable whether anything one could reasonably call 'black bile' was ever actually seen by a Graeco-Roman physician. Hippocrates and his followers did claim to see evidence of the black bile in dark faecal matter (probably due to congealed blood) and in darker than usual urine. But neither of these would actually have been black, nor is either of them properly speaking bile, which in living humans is only seen in vomit. One might accept the qualification that the Graeco-Roman physicians did not conceive of the humours as visible and tangible substances. It might make more sense to think of the humours as theoretical postulates that helped the ancient physicians to model the invisible processes underlying disease. But the difficulty still remains: the other three humours all had real, observable physiological correlates. Blood, bile, and phlegm are visible, tangible things – only black bile is not.

Black bile is also anomalous inasmuch as from the earliest records onwards it is evidently a disease, and not just a humour. As we saw in *Airs, Waters, Places*, Hippocrates used the term *melancholia* to identify a disease. By contrast, the other three humours have no disease that bears their name. There are diseases involving imbalances in the blood, phlegm, or bile, and diseases that cause disorders in these humours. But there is no disease called bloodiness, phlegminess, or biliousness; nor is there any disease caused solely by an excess of blood, phlegm, or bile (though bloodletting was a common treatment). A third problem is that it is by no means clear how we should interpret the physiology of the disease of melancholia in the earliest Graeco-Roman sources. To what real disease does melancholia, with its diversity of symptoms ranging from blackened urine to fear and sadness, actually correspond? Using modern disease categories, how would we diagnose the illness that the Greeks called melancholia? This has been the subject of much scholarly debate. The most plausible theory is that the physiological manifestations of melancholia correspond to the symptoms of black water fever, a complication of malaria, in which red blood cells burst in the urine causing it to turn dark red. This is all very tidy and plausible but it signally fails to do justice to the psychological symptoms of melancholia.

3   Melancholia hypochondriaca

The uncertain physiology of melancholia can be illustrated by the disease melancholia hypochondriaca. It began life in antiquity as a subspecies of melancholia with a specific location in the organs below the diaphragm. (The Greek *hypochondrion* designates the area immediately below the ribs and above the navel, containing the liver, the spleen, and so on; hence the later identification of melancholia hypochondriaca as 'the spleen'.) Galen found that in hypochondriac patients the normal symptoms of melancholia were associated with flatulence and impaired digestion.[4] It is not clear

---

[4] Stanley Jackson, 'Melancholia and the Waning of the Humoral Theory', *Journal of the History of Medicine* 33 (1978), 367–76 (at p. 367).

exactly when hypochondria began to take on its modern meaning of a 'preoccupation with having or acquiring a serious, undiagnosed medical illness'.[5] Elements of the modern meaning were available in the sixteenth century. In *The Anatomy of Melancholy* Burton says of this '*Hypocondriacall or flatuous melancholy*' that '*the symptomes are so ambiguous* saith Crato [Johannes Crato von Krafftheim, 1519–1585] in a counsell of his for a Noblewoman, *that the most exquisite Physitians cannot determine of the part affected.*'[6] The Swiss physician Felix Plater (1536–1614) records that patients with melancholia hypochondriaca complain of a large number of ailments. Some of these were no doubt due to an underlying melancholic illness, but others were merely imagined. The patient would imagine that every last little change in the body was a sign of serious illness, and would go through each part of the body from head to toe analysing its problems.[7] The seventeenth-century British physicians Thomas Willis and Thomas Sydenham separated hypochondriasis from melancholia proper, though they were unusual in doing so: for most early modern writers melancholia hypochondriaca remained part of or a stage in melancholia. 'The spleen' was normally just a synonym for melancholia.[8] In *A Treatise of the Hypochondriack and Hysterick Passions*, Bernard de Mandeville (1670–1733) distinguished between melancholia and hypochondria on the grounds that melancholia was a species of madness, while hypochondria was not. In other words, while melancholics suffered from delusions, hypochondriacs were merely assailed by doubts and fears: 'I'm grown peevish and fretfull, irresolute, suspicious, every thing offends me, and a trifle puts me in a Passion,' the hypochondriac might say.[9] Dissatisfied with the diagnosis from his physician, he would go from doctor to doctor, with each giving a different view – what is now known as 'doctor shopping'. In the classical tradition of melancholia we find an even earlier source for this apparently irrational behaviour towards physicians. Isḥāq ibn 'Imrān records that a melancholic will pester his physician and shower him with luxurious gifts, but when the physician gives advice, the patient will refuse to follow it. This, he claims, is a peculiarity found in all melancholics.[10]

If the behaviour of hypochondriacs was singular, the physiological symptoms of hypochondriasis were not that novel or unusual. They were all part of the traditional gamut of symptoms of melancholia.

[5] DSM-5, 315.   [6] Burton, *Anatomy*, vol. I, 410.

[7] Felix Plater, *Observationum, in hominis affectibus plerisq[ue], corpori et animo, functionum laesione, dolore, aliave molestia et vitio incommodantibus, libri tres* (Basel: Waldkirch, 1614), 70.

[8] So Boerhaave, cited by Jackson, *Melancholia*, 286.   [9] Jackson, *Melancholia*, 288.

[10] Isḥāq ibn 'Imrān, *Maqāla fī'l-mālīḫūliyā*, 28.

Mandeville was still persuaded that hypochondriasis originated in the abdomen. What we see in the history of hypochondriasis is a separating out or budding off of a syndrome that was originally part of melancholia but increasingly came to have its own distinct profile and aetiology, central to which was the patient's belief in an imagined ailment. Nicholas Robinson (1697–1775) confirmed of hypochondriacal patients that 'none knows what they feel and suffer'.[11] By 1800 at the latest, the diagnosis had settled in its modern form. William Cullen (1710–1790) observed that the false imaginings of hypochondriacs were confined to their state of health.[12]

A child of melancholia, hypochondriasis shared its parent's problematic nature. As we have seen, despite the elusiveness of melancholia's physiological basis, Greek physicians seem not to have doubted that it was real. Still, the elusiveness played out, if not in doubts about melancholia's existence, then in disagreement about its physiological aetiology. Where did it come from and in which organs did it manifest itself? What did the physical illness really consist of? These doubts and questions found a kind of answer in a disease, melancholia hypochondriaca, that gave voice precisely to the uncertainty concerning melancholia's physical nature. The hypochondriac compulsively asks a question, 'what's wrong with me?', that the physicians cannot answer with one voice. The diagnosis of hypochondriasis explains their failure to agree: there is in fact no disease. Hypochondriasis provides the physicians with an answer to what was unanswerable. The question 'what's wrong with me?' now becomes answerable by being turned back on the hypochondriac: 'what's wrong with you is that you keep on asking what's wrong with you'.

4　Rufus of Ephesus' *On Melancholia*

That is not to say that melancholia is utterly elusive. The underlying physiology might have been difficult to pin down, and the symptoms often hard to account for, but physicians in the Graeco-Roman tradition were able to diagnose melancholia with some confidence and reliability. They evidently had a clear and determinate notion of how melancholia presented and hence an answer (or a number of answers) to the question, 'what's wrong with me?' They also knew that melancholia occupied a clear conceptual space in their nosologies, between epilepsy and madness.[13] However, the nature and complex interrelations of the ancient textual sources make any attempt at a historical reconstruction of Graeco-Roman

---

[11] Jackson, *Melancholia*, 293.　[12] *Ibid.*, 299.
[13] Jouanna, 'At the Roots of Melancholy', 236.

melancholia, and hence any attempt to establish an original form of melancholia which a history of the subject might use as its starting point, highly problematic. The earliest evidence from the Hippocratic sources, though clear enough, is very slender. There is no Hippocratic treatise on melancholia, only scattered references and a small handful of case histories. The provenance of these sources is also unclear. The Hippocratic corpus was probably composed over an extended period by a number of writers. Galen's utterances on melancholia are almost certainly authentic, but they have their own problems. As Isḥāq ibn 'Imrān notes, Galen's statements on melancholia are scattered through his writings.[14] Moreover, they are either oddly tangential to the actual subject (*On the Affected Parts*) or are composites of other writers' ideas. Isolating a Hippocratic or Galenic theory of melancholia is made even harder by the schematizing and homogenizing effects of tradition, as we saw in the previous chapter. The unitary model of melancholia that we find in these later Graeco-Roman physicians seems to be a simplification of the tradition's origins.

In what follows I have taken a guardedly pragmatic approach. Rather than compiling a version of Graeco-Roman melancholia from the many and diverse ancient sources, I have privileged one version of the disorder. This is the account in Rufus of Ephesus' two books, *On Melancholia*. Rufus deserves his special status in the tradition for three reasons. First, in late antiquity and the Middle Ages, Rufus was accorded a very high status by medical writers, perhaps second only to the great Galen, and some even rated him Galen's equal.[15] On the subject of melancholia, however, there was no competition: Rufus' treatise *On Melancholia* was considered the best on the subject. 'Among the recent physicians, Rufus of Ephesus has composed the best work on melancholy,' wrote Galen himself.[16] Indeed, Galen's own account of melancholia relied heavily on Rufus, a debt that he acknowledged.[17] Not least because of his acknowledged excellence, Rufus occupies a unique position in the history of melancholia. Just as the Galenic view of melancholia derived largely from Rufus, so did the picture of melancholia in medieval Arabic texts. Isḥāq ibn 'Imrān said that the only satisfactory text on melancholia was by Rufus, and he based his own treatise on melancholia on Rufus.[18] And because medieval Western medicine derived chiefly from translated Arabic sources, it too was based on Rufus. Until the Renaissance Rufus

---

[14] Isḥāq ibn 'Imrān, *Maqāla fī'l-mālīḫūliyā*, 2.   [15] Pormann, 'Introduction', 27.
[16] *Ibid.*
[17] Michael W. Dols, *Majnūn: The Madman in Islamic Society* (Oxford University Press, 1992), 25–6.
[18] Isḥāq ibn 'Imrān, *Maqāla fī'l-mālīḫūliyā*, 1.

was the pre-eminent source on melancholia, whether or not he was acknowledged as such. Rufus' treatise has not survived in its entirety. All we have are quotations from Rufus, some attributed, some not, in Galen and other later writings (mainly in Arabic). These, especially the relevant passages from Isḥāq ibn ʿImrān, can be pieced together to form a fair overall picture of Rufus' theory, and they include a substantial amount of intriguing detail. But the picture is still incomplete, and it seems reasonable to supplement Rufus with the views of other classical and later writers where these helpfully fill the gaps.

Rufus' treatise is divided into two parts, but it is better thought of as dealing with four questions: the disease's causes, its development, its symptoms (all three of which form part one of Rufus' treatise), and its treatment (part two). The distinction between causes and development is untidy but important. Isḥāq ibn ʿImrān reports that Rufus 'singled out in his art one kind of this disease – namely, the hypochondriac illness – while omitting to discuss its other kinds'.[19] He later confirms this, adding that Rufus said his discussion of melancholia hypochondriaca was 'linked and connected to the other two types. Moreover, by my discussion of this one kind of melancholy, I hint at the other two types as regards the symptoms which I have listed and the treatment which I have described' (Rufus, 29). In other words, the symptoms and treatment of the three types would appear to be broadly the same, and so is the aetiology, so that Rufus' account of the one type is representative of all three. Galen seems to confirm this when he says that 'nothing is missing' in Rufus' treatise. On the other hand, the three types do differ, especially in respect of the development and severity of the disease. In order to bring the different types into focus, it makes sense to look at the disease's development separately.

5   Aetiology

According to Rufus, the aetiology of melancholia is relatively straightforward. It first appears as an overheating of the liver and stomach (Rufus, 31). Galen, by contrast, argues for a swelling of the portal vein in the liver. Others seem to have believed that a blockage in the mesenteric veins was responsible. But all the classical authorities agree that the location of the disease's first manifestation is in the hypochondria. Various indications support this: if relief is provided to the abdomen, the pain decreases; but if the abdomen becomes dry, the opposite occurs. Vomiting also provides

---

[19] Rufus, *On Melancholy*, 27. Subsequent references to this edition appear in the main texts in the form 'Rufus, 27'.

relief. The main cause would therefore appear to be indigestion (Rufus, 31).[20] Aëtius, in his summary of Rufus, states that this exogenous form of melancholia is the result of a bad diet. But there is also, so Rufus seems to say, an endogenous kind of melancholia that results from patients' 'nature and original mixture' (*physis kai hē ex archēs krasis*), presumably a constitutional excess of black bile or a tendency to overheating in hypochondria (Rufus, 35). It is worth noting that only very rarely in the ancient sources do we find a form of melancholia with purely psychological causes. Hippocrates reports the case of a woman of Thasos who was of a gloomy cast of mind 'after a grief with a reason for it'.[21] Aretaeus says that the symptoms can be purely psychological and the disease can present without any trace of black bile, but he maintains that even in such cases that have no physical symptoms, the aetiology is nonetheless physiological.[22] Later writers would contest this view and argue for a purely psychological causation. Burton provides a long list of psychological causes, including education, frights, insults, loss of liberty, poverty, and 'an Heape of other Accidents'.[23] From late antiquity into the early modern period, astrological influence was often cited, and supernatural causes of melancholia (God, the Devil, witches) were a part of the early modern Christian tradition.

6   Course

The disease develops into one of three types: general, encephalic, and hypochondriac.[24] In general melancholia, black bile spreads through the whole system. In the encephalic form, black bile gathers in the brain. In the earliest phase of the disease the only signs are psychological: 'fear, anxiety, suspicion aimed at one particular thing'. At first these symptoms are relatively mild, but they become more acute with time (Rufus, 37). It also seems that the psychological symptoms can themselves make the disease worse, in a kind of feedback loop. Indeed, this is a core feature of melancholia. The initial onset of the disease in the hypochondria gives rise to anxiety, and this in turn exacerbates the underlying disease, so that 'violent thoughts and worries make one succumb to melancholy'. The same is true of intense intellectual activity. Excessive thinking is

---

[20] So too Diocles: if the veins leading to stomach are heated, they can become blocked so that food is hard to digest (cited by Flashar, *Melancholie*, 50–1).

[21] *Epidemics*, III, xvii, 11, in *Hippocrates I*, 277.   [22] Flashar, *Melancholie*, 76–77.

[23] Burton, *Anatomy*, vol. I, 356.

[24] Although Rufus does not discuss these three and the specifics of their development, their presence in Galen suggests a source in Rufus: see Flashar, *Melancholie*, 92–3, and Rufus, 82.

dangerous (Rufus, 53), especially when focused on one area of study (Rufus, 47). Rufus records the case of a man whose melancholia was exacerbated by his obsession with geometry (Rufus, 69). There may in fact be a constitutional predisposition to melancholia in 'people of excellent nature' (Rufus, 47).

As for the physiological development of the disease, overheating in the hypochondria causes yellow bile to be burnt up, during which a patient will exhibit unruly behaviour. Only when the combustion of the bile is complete does a despondent phase ensue (Rufus, 35). As the disease develops it becomes more serious, because the black bile 'becomes inveterate'. The mood of the patient becomes fixed and resistant to therapy (Rufus, 37). When ulcers appear on the body, death is imminent (Rufus, 39). Equally ominous are ulcers in the intestines, which are revealed by blood in the faeces (Rufus, 43). Another acute development in later stages of melancholia is the onset of epilepsy or hemiplegia (paralysis of one side of the body: Rufus, 53). The former would become an established part of the pathogenesis of melancholia.

Seasonal variations can affect the course of the illness. As we saw in Chapter 1, Hippocrates thought that a dry northeast wind in late summer could cause bile to become black bile.[25] Rufus believes that autumn is a dangerous season, for it can cause bad digestion (Rufus, 47). And then, if the patient acquires 'bad blood' during the winter, in spring when the blood is stirred the black bile will spread through the body and to the brain in particular. This can result in melancholic 'pustules, abscesses, swellings, tumours, headaches', and other signs (Rufus, 45).

7   Symptoms

The differences between the types of melancholia are most apparent in their physical symptoms. Melancholia hypochondriaca gives rise to a litany of digestive complaints. Flatulence and a distended stomach are the key signs of this type, especially after eating foods that are hard to digest (Rufus, 50). Indigestion and flatulence are particularly common among the elderly, who are especially prone to melancholia 'since the old are naturally depressed' (Rufus, 39). A distinctive symptom is pricking pains in the abdomen (Rufus, 73), 'similar to ants moving' (Rufus, 65). Melancholia sometimes reveals itself in black bodily discharges, whether vomit or faeces or urine. But this is not the case in every melancholic: 'rather, phlegm appears most frequently' (Rufus, 41). Skin problems

---

[25] Flashar, *Melancholie*, 21–2.

include ulcers, 'dull-white leprosy', pimples, and mange, as well as bleeding haemorrhoids (Rufus, 41).

Encephalic melancholia can be experienced as lightness of the head, which is caused by *pneuma* rising to the brain (Rufus, 33). Also associated with the effects of *pneuma* are protuberant eyes and thick lips. The skin of melancholics may also turn black (Rufus, 35). They have little hair (Rufus, 37). 'Their movements are powerful and quick, and they can do nothing slowly', again because of the *pneuma* (Rufus, 39). (These may also be symptoms of general melancholia, or indeed physical characteristics of the melancholy temperament. Physical appearance would later become a key feature of the humoral theory, whether connected with illness or just a relatively healthy preponderance of one humour, as, for instance, in the 'lean and hungry look' of the melancholic Cassius in Shakespeare's *Julius Caesar*.) Hippocrates records episodes of lisping, loss of speech, and stammering.[26] Rufus also identifies speech impairment as a symptom of melancholia: 'they generally speak fast, they lisp, and stammer, since they cannot control their tongue' (Rufus, 35).

The core psychological symptoms of melancholia were established by Hippocrates. 'If the fear and despondency last for a long time, that is the melancholic state.'[27] It is these symptoms that have given the tradition of melancholia a 'remarkable consistency', in the words of Stanley Jackson. In fact, a wide range of symptoms is recorded, but by far the most common are fear and sadness of long duration and without evident cause. We have seen that the lack of any evident cause is a defining feature of melancholia hypochondriaca. The lack of an evident cause is connected to the disorder's long duration: there appears to be no reason why the fear and sadness do not end, as they would if the symptoms had a determinate cause, such as mourning the death of a friend or relative. So the patient feels the need to keep asking 'what's wrong with me?' (The similarities and differences between melancholia and mourning were a subject of discussion long before Freud's 1917 essay 'Mourning and Melancholia'.) The compulsive return to this question is one of the defining features of melancholia.

Another notable feature of melancholia is the place it accords to fear and anxiety. And there are other behavioural symptoms. The woman of Thasos in the Hippocratic *Epidemics* suffered from 'coma ... aversion to food, despondency, sleeplessness, irritability, restlessness [*dysphoriai*], the

---

[26] For lisping and loss of speech, see *Epidemics*, II, v, 1, in *Hippocrates VII*, trans. by Wesley D. Smith, Loeb Classical Library (Cambridge, MA: Harvard University Press), 75. For stammering, see *Epidemics*, II, vi, 1, in *Hippocrates VII*, 81.

[27] *Hippocrates IV*, 185.

mind being affected by melancholia'.[28] Strange and terrifying dreams are typical.[29] In Rufus the psychological symptoms become more specific and perplexing. 'The beginning of melancholy is indicated by fear, anxiety, and suspicion aimed at one particular thing' (Rufus, 37). Anxiety is stronger in women who experience 'repugnant fantasies' (Rufus, 39), presumably of a sexual nature. Aretaeus claims that lovesickness is a symptom of melancholia.[30] A melancholic's fear might relate to family members or to humans at large (Rufus, 33). Some fear thunder (Rufus, 37), others drowning (Rufus, 71). Some melancholics will fear what is good for them and crave harmful things. It is common for melancholics to crave solitude (Rufus, 37). Unsurprisingly, suicide is reported, whether out of a desire to escape some greater evil or because they imagine 'it is beautiful to die, like some barbarians' (Rufus, 33–5). Some 'ardently desire to discuss death' (Rufus, 37). Galen, perhaps following Epicurus, says that some melancholics combine a fear of death with a death wish.[31] Immoderate anger and violence are also recorded. When emboldened by the overheating of yellow bile, 'they brawl and commit the most outrageous acts' (Rufus, 35). There are specific obsessions (e.g. cleanliness) and aversions (particular foods or drinks or animals). Central to Rufus' understanding of melancholia is the presence of delusions. At a low level the melancholic might suffer from an unfavourable opinion of himself (Rufus, 71). One of the charms of the literature on melancholia is the recording of more bizarre delusions, often of a physical nature. One melancholic believed he had swallowed a viper (Rufus, 37). Another thought his body was made of clay, one that he had no head, and another that his skin was made of parchment (Rufus, 33).

8   Treatment

One of the most persuasive features of Greek medicine is the neat fit between pathology and treatment. Different physical and psychological treatments are recommended for different types and phases of the disease, and they are carefully matched. The underlying aim of most of the physiological treatments was to purge or purify the bodily system, and even where treatments aim at other effects, such as stimulation or pain relief, purging usually plays a part. Psychological treatments are generally directed at the alleviation of fear and sadness by improving the patient's mood or altering his thought processes.

[28] *Epidemics*, III, xvii, 2, in *Hippocrates I*, 263.
[29] Hippocrates, *De morbis*, cited by Flashar, *Melancholie*, 51.
[30] Flashar, *Melancholie*, 78–9.   [31] *Ibid.*, 106.

The first and most immediate need is to provide relief for the hypochondria by evacuating the bowels. Evacuation by vomiting can be induced by emetics such as radish, origany, and thyme. But Rufus adds a word of caution: the use of emetics should be moderated, as their excessive use can actually make the illness worse (Rufus, 49). Mint decoctions help by expelling wind. True germander and ground pine promote urination and relieve indigestion (Rufus, 55). The stomach can also be treated externally. Heating the epigastric region with warm compresses (Rufus, 51) or covering with blankets is recommended (Rufus, 59). Trapped wind can be reduced by the laying on of bandages dressed with seeds that dissolve wind, such as mustard. Alternatively one can anoint the belly with oil of lily. Rufus also recommends the use of cupping glasses to relieve the stomach (Rufus, 53).

Numerous preparations are recommended to purge the system and so reduce the concentration of noxious black bile. These include epithyme and aloe (Rufus, 49), absinth juice, colocynth juice, and black hellebore (Rufus, 51). At more advanced stages of the disease the system can be purged by bloodletting (Rufus, 65).

All Greek physicians advise the regulation of the diet, both solid and liquid. It is important to eat well, which means avoiding heavy and indigestible food. Healthy foods for melancholics include semolina bread, chicken and kite meat, and small rockfish. The patient should aim to put on a moderate amount of weight. White wine in moderation is helpful, as is thick vinegar before bedtime (Rufus, 51). Wine should not be taken in excess, but rather little and often. Used in this way, wine 'delights the soul and cleanses it of sadness' (Rufus, 61). Tepid water is good after a meal as it aids in the 'expulsion of superfluities through urine and faeces from all the pores of the body' (Rufus, 59).

Some physical treatments are designed to address the psychological symptoms, whether by acting directly on the brain or by lifting the mood through stimulation. This was also the aim of a range of psychological treatments. The best and most celebrated of all remedies is the 'holy remedy' (*hiera*), a mixture of many herbs and spices administered with honeyed water and salt. The specific efficacy of *hiera* in treating melancholia is that 'by removing most things from the head it is beneficial to reasoning' (Rufus, 55–7), though it also acts as a purgative. Light exercise, especially walking, has a positive effect (Rufus, 51). Rufus also claims that sexual intercourse reduces the hot passions and makes the temper milder (Rufus, 61). Psychological cures can alleviate the melancholic mood or even prevent it developing at all. A rapid intervention can hide from the patient the true nature of his illness: if the patient can be persuaded that he is only suffering from indigestion, the psychological effects of the disease can be mitigated (Rufus, 53). Once the melancholic mood has set in, the patient should be protected against excessive belief, terror, joy, and cogitation. Diversions and distractions can help. Long and extended journeys provide distraction and amusement (Rufus, 51). Deep sadness can be relieved by amusements such as music (Rufus, 69). Soranus suggests the theatre.[32]

It is worth dwelling on the thought that the psychological symptoms of melancholia become worse once the patient is aware of the diagnosis. What exactly is meant by this? Why should the diagnosis itself have an adverse effect on the patient's state of mind? One possibility is that the disease is known to be extremely grave and the prognosis for patients very poor. Knowledge of such a grave diagnosis might well send the patient into a deep depression. This effect is well documented in modern medicine, notably in the depressive effects of receiving a diagnosis of cancer. According to the US National Cancer Institute, depression affects between 15 and 25 per cent of cancer patients.[33] If this explanation were correct, one would expect Rufus to say that the psychological impact of the diagnosis was grief, fear, and similar emotions, but in fact Rufus refers to a wider range of cognitive symptoms. This is what Rufus says (or what ar-Rāzī in his *Comprehensive Book* says that Rufus says): 'Do not make the patient suspect that he has melancholy. Rather just treat him for indigestion; help him against his excessive belief, terror and joy; and keep him from [too much] thinking' (Rufus, 53). One would expect a patient to respond to the news of a terminal prognosis with grief and anxiety; 'belief', 'joy', and excessive thinking do not sound like responses to a terminal diagnosis. Instead, Rufus seems to be listing specific psychological symptoms of melancholia. These symptoms represent a phase in the pathogenesis of the disease. The disease begins in the 'hypochondries' (organs immediately below the diaphragm) but spreads to the brain and causes turbulent emotional and cognitive symptoms ('belief', 'joy', and excessive thinking). By concealing the diagnosis of melancholia, the physician can perhaps prevent the disease from entering this dangerous phase – dangerous because once it begins the patient is prone to a continuous feedback loop of worsening symptoms. The more turbulent your mental state is, the worse the symptoms of melancholia become, because you become anxious and alarmed about your own condition. In other words, Rufus suggests a link between the psychopathology of melancholia and self-consciousness. The phenomenon he alludes to bears some similarity to the modern notion of rumination. As we noted in the introduction, rumination – the tendency to

---

[32] *Ibid.*, 83.
[33] www.cancer.gov/cancertopics/pdq/supportivecare/depression/Patient/page2

focus rigidly on one's own depression – is a common symptom of depression and a major obstacle to recovery. In fact, there is a tradition linking ancient melancholy rumination with modern depressive rumination: in *As You Like It*, the melancholic Jaques complains that 'my often *rumination* wraps me in a most humorous sadness' (Act IV, scene i).[34]

9   Medieval and early modern physiological paradigms

The repertoire of herbal and other preparations (or *materia medica*, as it had been known since the first century AD) saw a considerable expansion in the hands of the medieval Arab physicians and later medieval medicine. Indeed, this growth was the major contribution of the Middle Ages to the medicine of melancholia. It went hand in hand with a growth in sympathetic medicine. The sympathetic system was based on the notion that the curative properties of a substance derived their efficacy from some similarity, whether visual or verbal or analogical, between it and the illness or the affected part. This kind of thinking, while not entirely alien to Ancient Greek notions of the properties of substances (cold, dry, wet, warm), was chiefly the result of the growth of magical and astrological thinking in the Middle Ages.

The early modern period saw the beginnings of more significant shifts in the physiological underpinnings of the theory of melancholia. As we saw in the case of Rufus and the other Greek physicians, the specifics of aetiology, pathogenesis, symptoms, and therapies were to a great extent dependent on the underlying physiological paradigms. One way of telling the story of melancholia (and depression) is in terms of these physiological paradigms. The details of the practice of medicine in a given time and place make sense within (and only within) a set of wider beliefs about the world. Graeco-Roman medicine was based on a belief that the constitution of the body is affected by environmental influences, and this was a given even for medics who did not adhere to a strict Galenic humoral theory. Along with the belief in environmental influences went an assumption that most illnesses are systemic in origin, even if they only affected one part of the body, and could therefore be treated with a systemic regimen. It was this historically specific overarching mentality that gave meaning to the particular symptoms and therapies and the causal mechanisms that purportedly connected them. In a similar way the symptomatology of modern depression and the magic-bullet psycho-pharmaceuticals prescribed by our doctors depend for their meaning on a

---

[34] William Shakespeare, *As You Like It*, ed. Agnes Latham, The Arden Shakespeare (London: Routledge, 1996), 95.

broadly Kraepelinian model of mental illness and more specifically on the assumption that emotional and cognitive states are a function of brain chemistry.

This picture of a close and necessary correlation between medical practice on the ground and large-scale features of scientific theory is, needless to say, a simplification. For one thing, it is not the case that historical change in medicine is driven by changing theoretical paradigms. If it were, then we should expect to see high-level theoretical change moving ahead of empirical science and necessarily dragging the latter in its wake.[35] The specifics of aetiology, pathogenesis, symptoms, and therapies would thereafter gradually fall into line with the new scientific paradigm. In reality things are messier. Change in the theory of melancholia was both slower and less even than the paradigm-shift view would suggest. Some traditional elements such as lycanthropy proved remarkably persistent, surviving on the oxygen of authority alone. Other traditional elements might survive a paradigm shift for no other reason than that they were (or were believed to be) empirically warranted. This is obviously the case for the psychology of melancholia. The remarkably persistent core definition – fear and anger of long duration and without evident cause – is not dependent in any obvious way on the Greek or any subsequent physiological paradigm. (Quite why it proved so persistent will concern us in Chapters 4 and 5.) It is also the case that some elements of the physiology of melancholia proved remarkably stubborn and hard to shift. Melancholia never consisted of a single body of theory; it consisted of a number of discrete but interlinked theoretical objects, which could change independently from and out of sync with one another.

10   Mechanical and hydraulic theories

Paradigm shifts are rarely identifiable as such at the time. The first significant break with Galenic humoralism was a model based on mechanical and hydraulic explanations. This can be seen as part of a larger shift in science away from an Aristotelian style of physics based on the qualities inherent in substances, towards a Cartesian-Newtonian science based on numerical quantities that could be measured and related to one another in mathematical formulae. It was implicit in this quantitative model that the four humours were now defunct, since the humours were grounded in qualitative reasoning. Thus, the Swiss physician Albrecht von Haller (1708–1777) argued that there are not in fact four qualitatively distinct

---

[35] See Thomas S. Kuhn, *The Structure of Scientific Revolutions* (University of Chicago Press, 1962).

humours, but 'numberless degrees' of quantitatively different bodily constitutions. Melancholia was to be categorized by quantity, not quality.[36] However, the ultimate victory of the quantitative physiology was very slow in coming.

In physiology the Cartesian-Newtonian idea of science first expressed itself in a model based on the dynamics of fluids circulating around the body. Metaphors of fluid movement were already in use to describe melancholia in the early seventeenth century. To some extent the hydraulic model merely elevated these metaphors into scientific theory.[37] One of the pioneers of the iatromechanical school was Friedrich Hoffmann (1660–1742). In Hoffmann's account of melancholia, the psychological symptoms are still essentially the same as they were for Rufus: the fixing of attention on a single idea; anxiety, dejection, and irritability; a love of solitude. The physical symptoms, however, have changed somewhat. In tune with his model of fluid dynamics, Hoffmann identifies a small, weak pulse, 'deep and laborious' breathing, and a pale face as symptomatic. These are all signs that the movement of fluids round the body has slowed dangerously. In a more traditional vein, the melancholic suffers from a voracious appetite, uncomfortable abdomen, and acrid urine.[38] The cause of melancholia is 'a retardation of the circulation', though this is only the proximate cause: the original causes are long grief or fear, too much sex, diseases, abuse of alcohol or drugs, 'a preternatural afflux of blood to the brain', 'gross foods', or a sedentary lifestyle.[39] (The sedentary life became a preoccupation of physicians in the early modern period; this was entirely in conformity with earlier Galenic theory, but it became more prominent in the context of the iatromechanists' emphasis on the poor circulation of the blood in melancholia.) Different fluids had different physical properties, notably speed and density, and when a fluid's composition changed, its dynamics would also change. In melancholia the body fluid turned acidic and fixed, and its motions became sluggish, resulting in despondency. Melancholia could also change the composition of the blood, making it warmer, heavier, and darker than normal.[40] Like the Graeco-Roman medical writers, Hoffmann recommends treatments for both mind and body. Peruvian (cinchona) bark, an example of the expansion of the *materia medica* thanks to the colonial

---

[36] Albrecht von Haller, *First Lines of Physiology*, 2 vols. (Edinburgh: Elliot, 1786), vol. I, 89; first published as *Elementa physiologiae corporis humani* (Lausanne: Bousquet, 1757).

[37] Kutzer, *Anatomie*, 120–1.

[38] Friedrich Hoffmann, *A System of the Practice of Medicine*, 2 vols. (London: Murray, 1783), vol. II, 298–9; first published as *Medicina rationalis systematica*, 4 vols. in 9 (Halle: Renger, 1718–34).

[39] Hoffmann, *System*, vol. II, 300.   [40] *Ibid.*, 299.

trade, 'raises the pulse and spirits'.[41] It should be accompanied by
'exercise and the drinking of warm liquors'.[42] Bloodletting was still
practised to thin the blood and improve its circulation.[43] Similar effects
could be achieved with moderately warm baths and mineral waters.[44]
('Taking the waters' was another fashion of the early modern period.)
Also recommended were moderate exercise, cheerful conversation,
water mixed with one-quarter Rhine wine, and 'the visceral elixir, with
tincture of orange peel'.[45]

The greatest authority of eighteenth-century medicine, Herman
Boerhaave (1668–1738), likewise applied a theory based on fluid dynamics. He viewed black bile, much like Rufus, as a pathogenic material that
was not, however, qualitatively different from the other fluids, but
resulted from mechanical or hydrodynamic actions.[46] It came about
through the expulsion of the naturally highly movable parts of the
blood and the fixing of the heavier, less mobile parts: 'then will the
Blood become thick, black, fat, and earthy. And this defect will be
call'd by the name of an *Atribiliar Humor*, or *Melancholy Juyce*.'[47] The
symptoms were the same as those reported by Hoffmann; like him,
Boerhaave considered slowing of circulation as the proximate cause of
despondency of mood. In the early stages of the disease, when the blood
had not yet fully thickened, psychological therapies might be effective. The
physician should offer patients a variety of objects for their attention,
without, of course, letting them know that it was a treatment at all.
(Deception of this kind would become a common theme, not only in
medical practice but also in literature and especially theatre. Again the
rationale was to direct patients' consciousness away from their own
sickly self; self-consciousness was as great an enemy as melancholia.)
Beyond this, treatments belonged to the traditional categories: good
sleep, moist air, light foods, and 'wholesome Liquors'. The most effica-
cious treatments involved the use of 'diluting Medicines' to improve
blood flow: fruit juices, broths, and mineral water.[48] But if the disease
had progressed, the emphasis should be on laxatives.[49] The final, incura-
ble stages of the disease were characterized by putrefaction and the
'gangrenous eating of all the abdominal entrails'. Now all the physician
could do was prescribe opium as a palliative.[50]

[41] *Ibid.*, vol. I, 7.   [42] *Ibid.*, 8.   [43] *Ibid.*, 10.   [44] *Ibid.*, II, 69.   [45] *Ibid.*, 129.
[46] Jackson, *Melancholia*, 119.
[47] Herman Boerhaave, *Practical Aphorisms* (London: Cowse, 1715), 291; first published as
Aphorismi de cognoscendis et curandis morbis, in usum doctrinae domesticae (Leiden: van der
Linden, 1715).
[48] *Ibid.*, 293.   [49] *Ibid.*, 296.   [50] *Ibid.*, 298.

11   Nerve-based theories

In the course of the eighteenth century the focus shifted away from hydraulics and towards the nerves. Some believed the nerves to be hollow vessels filled with a vital 'aetherial' fluid, an adaptation of Newton's notion of an ethereal substance that he held responsible for the action of gravity. Others believed that the nerves were chords subject to vibration and tension. Only with Galvani's discovery of bioelectricity in the 1770s, specifically the fact that electricity could power muscle movement in frogs' legs, did the idea gain ground that the nerves conducted electrical impulses.

The idea of nervous sensibility moved forward on a broad scientific and cultural front, in novels as well as medicine. The medical theory of William Cullen (1710–1790) reflects this shift. Cullen's description of the melancholic temperament emphasizes sensibility and pays correspondingly less attention to the traditional elements of anger, fear, and irritability. Melancholics are characterized by 'sensibility, frequently exquisite, but with great accuracy; moderate irritability, with remarkable tenacity of impressions'.[51] Some new physical symptoms are cited, but most belong to the traditional repertoire, including 'diseases, (of the veins,) haemorrhoids, apoplexy, cachexy, obstructions of the viscera, particularly of the liver, dropsies, affections of the alimentary canal'. Ultimately, these are all attributed to 'slower and weaker influence of the nervous power'.[52] That is to say, allowing for some shifts of emphasis, the symptoms of melancholia remain broadly within the Graeco-Roman tradition, even though the cause of melancholia, an underlying nervous weakness, is quite new.

In Cullen, the beginnings of another shift in emphasis can also be seen, from sensibility to debility. Eighteenth-century culture had created a self-appointed aristocracy of sensibility. The good, the true, and (especially) the beautiful were to be felt as much as known. Not for the first time, the diseases of sensitivity – melancholia, hypochondria, the spleen, 'the vapours' – became fashionable. Some physicians were critical of the extent to which medicine was driven by fashion. In 1786 the Inverness doctor James Makittrick Adair (1728–1802) published his highly critical *Essays on Fashionable Diseases*, which went through three editions. Within a few years the star of sensibility would begin to wane. In Britain the alarming shockwaves of the French Revolution saw to it that sensibility, with its connotations of irrational and spontaneous enthusiasm, became politically suspect.

[51] William Cullen, *Lectures on the Materia Medica* (London: Lowndes, 1773), 18.
[52] Cullen, *Lectures*, 18–19.

After the revolution it might still be acceptable for women to be melancholy, but less so for men. And diseases of the nerves would increasingly be understood in terms of debility, not sensitivity. The nineteenth century would see a move towards diagnoses of asthenia, which were marked by strong gender differences. On one side stood the post-revolutionary ideal of mastery of the emotions and immunity to melancholia. Although women were encouraged to aspire to this ideal, it was clearly male gendered. On the other side was (predominantly female) weakness and emotionalism. Constitutional weakness being, so ancient prejudice would have it, more typical of women, the answer to the question 'what's wrong with me?' might well depend on your gender. And while the gendering of debility is most striking in the nineteenth century, it is reasonable to suppose that throughout its history the possibilities for experiencing melancholia have been different for women and men to some degree. Gendering, then, is a further complicating social factor in the history of melancholia and a major challenge to psychiatric realism. In the next chapter we will consider how and why the gendering of melancholia arises: of what kind is this gendering, where does it come from, and how deep does it go?

3   Melancholy men, depressed women?

1   The incidence of depression and melancholia by gender

The notebooks of the Buckinghamshire physician Sir Richard Napier (1607–1676) provide a rich insight into medical practice in seventeenth-century England. Napier's notes on 2,039 cases of mental disorders have survived, including many cases of melancholia.[1] One striking feature of these cases is that female melancholics outnumber male melancholics by around two to one.[2] Some 350 years after Napier made his notes the situation has not changed. In modern Western societies women are twice as likely to suffer from depression as men.[3] Why is there such a clear gender imbalance in the prevalence of melancholia and depression? Napier recorded that his female patients seemed to suffer from more unhappiness in their domestic and married lives. Perhaps this explains their higher rates of melancholia. Because of their subordinate position in society, women have traditionally been exposed to many potentially depressogenic stressors, not least among which are the burdens of menial work and caring for children, subordination to male social and political power, and the perceived and real obstacles to developing any kind of autonomous existence such as a career. A survey of depression in US college students appears to bear this out. In the relatively liberal environment of higher education, most of these depressogenic factors are absent: women students generally do not have families to support, and they enjoy greater equality of opportunity than women in society at large. Unsurprisingly, the results of the survey showed that female and male college students have roughly the same rates of depression: the gender imbalance seems to disappear.[4]

---

[1] Michael MacDonald, *Mystical Bedlam: Madness, Anxiety, and Healing in Seventeenth-Century England* (Cambridge University Press, 1981), 35.

[2] *Ibid.*, 36–40.

[3] Myrna Weissman *et al.*, 'Cross-National Epidemiology of Major Depression and Bipolar Disorder', *Journal of the American Medical Association* 276 (1996), 293–9.

[4] Susan Nolen-Hoeksema, *Sex Differences in Depression* (Stanford University Press, 1990), 26–8.

76

This is all eminently plausible, but possibly wrong. It may be that the US college survey was an anomaly. Or perhaps the incidence of depression among female students is lower because depressed women are less likely to make it to college in the first place. As for the apparently higher incidence of depression among women in society at large, the subordinate role of women is not as persuasive an explanation as it first seems. The problem is this. Assuming that high rates of depression in women are due to their subordinate roles, we would expect rates of depression among women to fall as social inequality is reduced. In fact the opposite has happened. Over the last fifty years in the West, women's status in society, measured in terms of education and income, has improved dramatically, but during the same period rates of depression among women have trebled. The social explanation, at least in the admittedly rather simplistic form in which I have framed it here, does not work. Of course, it may be that women are subject to some less obvious, more insidious social pressures. Alternatively, the high incidence of depression among women may have nothing to do with social forces. Perhaps, retrograde step though this may be, we should be asking whether women's psychology and physiology is responsible for their higher susceptibility to depression. For instance, there are specific forms of depression to which, by virtue of their physiology, only women are prone, such as post-natal depression, premenstrual depression, and menopausal depression. On their own these may not be sufficient to explain women's higher rates of depression, but they may be part of the picture.

In other words, the similar gender imbalance revealed by Napier's cases and modern epidemiology could be interpreted as confirmation of Jackson's continuity thesis. Perhaps women just *are* twice as likely to suffer from melancholia and depression. Most people will quite rightly be troubled by the suggestion that women are by nature more prone to depression than men. The idea becomes less obnoxious if we reverse the perspective. Instead of saying that women are by nature more prone to depression than men, we could say that depression is by its nature more likely to afflict women. This might not at first seem any better, but if we treat depression as a socially constructed belief and not as a natural kind, the obnoxiousness disappears. Instead of saying that women naturally fall into the category of depression, we might say that the category of depression has been constructed in such a way as to fit women better than men. In other words, the fact that women seem twice as likely to suffer from depression as men might not be a fact about women but a fact about the social construct depression. Post-natal and the other forms of specifically female depression might provide evidence for this. Traditionally these problems have been viewed as part of the general medical picture of depression, but why should they be? DSM-IV-TR placed the post-partum syndrome under the category of depression. The only thing that distinguishes post-partum depression from ordinary depression is that its onset is triggered within four weeks of giving birth. In all other respects the symptoms 'do not differ from the symptoms in non-post-partum mood episodes' (so DSM-IV-TR).[5] This would suggest that women suffering post-natal depression should be treated like other clinically depressed patients, presumably with a regime of antidepressant drugs and therapy. It is hard to see how the medicalization of post-natal depression could be of benefit to women. And it is easy to see how it could be prejudicial to them. It implies, for instance, that something in the physiology of women is *naturally* depressive. It is a stigma pure and simple. And the psychiatrists seem to have noticed this. In an appendix to DSM-IV-TR, 'premenstrual dysphoric disorder' is proposed as a separate syndrome and not part of depression. This seems to be a recognition on the part of the psychiatric profession that lumping specifically female health issues together with the disease of depression was detrimental to women and set back the cause of equal rights and equality of treatment for women. However, DSM-5 reinstated premenstrual dysphoric disorder as a subcategory of depression.[6]

In fact, the issue of gender bias in mental health is much wider than this. Different mental illnesses have different gender biases. Women are more likely to suffer from panic disorders and eating disorders. Men seem to suffer higher rates of autism, attention-deficit/hyperactivity disorder, and alcoholism. In some cases (e.g. alcoholism) a link between the disease and social conditions seems probable. In others (e.g. male autism), social causation is less likely. It may just be that the way we have chopped up mental disorders into kinds has led to a whole slew of unobvious gender biases.

So the gender bias in the prevalence of melancholia is one of the strongest challenges to the psychiatric realism on which Jackson's continuity thesis is based. The most plausible explanation for the seemingly consistent way in which disease constructs have skewed the prevalence of melancholia is that melancholia is a socially constructed belief. A significant body of historical work on melancholia supports this view, for it seems to show that the very concept melancholia is strongly gendered. However, in this chapter I will argue that the case for gendered social construction is by no means proven. There are four reasons for scepticism. First, although some historians of the early modern period have

---

[5] DSM-IV-TR, 422.   [6] DSM-5, 171–5.

argued that melancholia is gendered, they have argued that it is *male* gendered. But if melancholia is male gendered, why did Napier find twice as many melancholy women as men? Second, the 2:1 bias in the prevalence of melancholia turns out not to be a consistent picture. Third, while it would be quixotic to argue that there is no gendering in the construction of melancholia – indeed, there is bountiful evidence of it – the evidence is hugely variable in kind. The explanations for gendering given by the medical writers themselves or by historians show no consistent patterns. Fourth, the gendering of melancholia is often a misleading appearance. In many cases what is in fact gendered is a neighbouring concept such as reproductive physiology or the idea of genius. Often the strongest gendering effects emanate not from melancholia itself, but from other concepts that come into contact with it.

When we bring the long history of melancholia into view, the 2:1 gender bias breaks down and a more complex picture emerges. Since 1800 the picture does seem relatively consistent. Esquirol considered melancholia to be a predominantly female disorder.[7] Kraepelin believed that his version of melancholia, 'manic-depressive insanity', was more common in women than men.[8] In the early modern period the picture is less conclusive, despite the evidence of Napier's case records. Historians of early modern melancholia are not unanimous: one concludes that women were marginally more likely to suffer than men,[9] but another finds no evidence that melancholia was gendered.[10] To be sure, early modern melancholia had its equivalent of post-partum depression. Certain subtypes of melancholia were either confined to or more prevalent among women. Burton has a chapter on 'Maides, Nunnes, and Widowes Melancholy'.[11] In the 1623 edition of his *Treatise on Lovesickness* – love had been recognized as a cause of melancholia at least since Aretaeus in the first century AD – Jacques Ferrand claims that women are more susceptible than men.[12] In antiquity the picture is a little clearer, though the underlying reasons for it are not. Aretaeus argues that adult men are especially prone to the disease.[13] (All ancient authorities seem to agree that age is more important

[7] Jennifer Radden, *The Nature of Melancholy: From Aristotle to Kristeva* (New York: Oxford University Press, 2000), 42.

[8] Jackson, *Melancholia*, 192.

[9] Angus Gowland, 'The Problem of Early Modern Melancholy', *Past and Present* 191 (2006), 77–120 (at p. 99).

[10] H. C. Erik Midelfort, *A History of Madness in Sixteenth-Century Germany* (Stanford University Press, 1999), 6–7.

[11] Burton, *Anatomy*, vol. I, 414–18.

[12] Noga Arikha, *Passions and Tempers: A History of the Humours* (New York: Ecco, 2007), 162–4.

[13] Jackson, *Melancholia*, 40.

than gender: the mature or the old are much more prone to melancholia than the young.) Galen states that melancholia is more prevalent among men but more acute in women,[14] a view that derives from Rufus,[15] who states that anxiety is stronger in women and that they have lurid sexual fantasies.[16]

2   The gendering of physiology in melancholia

Thus far I have focused on the 2:1 bias towards women, but prevalence in the population is not the only way that gendering expresses itself. It can also show in variances of the acuteness of the disease and the character of its symptoms. In some sources male and female melancholia appear to be qualitatively different from one another. This may reflect the way disease categories have been cut up, or it may be that the attention of physicians is drawn more strongly to some phenomena than to others. More often it seems to be the result of the gendering of underlying physiological models. The most influential physiological theory in the history of Western medicine has without doubt been Aristotle's, and it is gendered to the point of misogyny. Aristotle argues that woman is created by means of an act of insemination that has not been carried through to completion. The nature of the child is carried in the father's seed. This semen is naturally hot, and when its heat is fully preserved during insemination into the receiving female body, a male child is produced. But if the natural heat of the male semen is cooled during insemination, for which various factors may be responsible such as climate or imperfect insemination, the child will be female.[17] Women are therefore the result of an imperfectly completed process. By analogy, women themselves are imperfect versions of men: 'the nature of man is the most rounded off and complete', Aristotle concludes in his *History of Animals*.[18] Psychological consequences naturally follow from the physiology. Women are softer, more complex, more emotional; men more straightforward, more 'spirited'. Women seem more susceptible to melancholia than men as they are 'more prone to despondency and less hopeful'.[19]

---

[14] Stanley Jackson, 'Galen – On Mental Disorders', *Journal of the History of the Behavioral Sciences* 5 (1969), 365–84 (at p. 375).

[15] Jackson, *Melancholia*, 36.   [16] Rufus, *On Melancholy*, 39.

[17] Aristotle, *De Generatione Animalium*, 766b15–17, in *The Complete Works of Aristotle: The Revised Oxford Translation*, ed. Jonathan Barnes, 2 vols., Bollingen Series LXXI (Princeton University Press, 1984), vol. I, 1186.

[18] Aristotle, *Historia Animalium*, 608b6–8, in *Complete Works*, vol. I, 949; compare Juliana Schiesari, *The Gendering of Melancholia: Feminism, Psychoanalysis, and the Symbolics of Loss in Renaissance Literature* (Ithaca, NY: Cornell University Press, 1992), 108.

[19] Aristotle, *Historia Animalium*, 608b11–12, in *Complete Works*, vol. I, 949.

Aristotle was crowned the king of philosophers in the Islamic and Christian Middle Ages – indeed, he was often referred to simply as 'the Philosopher' – though physicians did not always accept his dominance. They could and did derive quite different models of melancholia directly from the medical sources available to them in the translations and digests of Galen and Rufus. In particular, medical writers on melancholia seem not to have taken up Aristotle's argument that women are more prone to despondency than men. And, as a whole, Graeco-Roman medicine shows great diversity on the subject of gender, with different physiological models predicting that either men or women are more prone to melancholia or suffer more acutely from it. As we saw in Chapter 1, the qualities of bodies consisted in the mixtures of humours. Accordingly, in Graeco-Roman medicine, there is a spectrum of gender physiology, not a strict 'either/or' dualism.[20] Galen holds that men tend to be warmer and drier, and women are colder and moister. Men therefore have a greater tendency towards the bilious and hence the melancholic, while women tend towards the phlegmatic.[21] In the pseudo-Galenic *On the Sperm*, a different explanation is given. The hot and moist right side of the womb produces male children, the dry and cold left side female children, making women more prone to melancholia.[22] But again the picture is confused. In the pseudo-Galenic *Medical Definitions*, the author asks whether women have the same sexual physiology as men, and the answer is unambiguously 'yes': 'the female has the same [sexual] desire and shares the same diseases'.[23] According to this canonical text, there is in essence no difference between male and female melancholia or the underlying male and female physiology that generates it. The Aristotelian physiology may have been strongly biased against women; other Graeco-Roman physiologies were not or were less obviously biased.

3   Markedness and other forms of gendering

Less obvious forms of bias do indeed lurk behind this unexpected picture of a relatively ungendered physiology. These biases are structural in nature. As we saw in Chapter 1, Galenic medicine was highly rationalistic and systematic. It was grounded in a systematic understanding of the ways that bodies function, in which speculative reasoning involving resemblance and analogy play at least as large a part as empirical observation. At the centre of this system is an idealized image of the human body,

---

[20] Diarmaid MacCulloch, *The Reformation* (New York: Viking, 2004), 610–11.
[21] Schöner, *Viererschema*, 91.   [22] Arikha, *Passions*, 81–2.
[23] Flemming, *Medicine*, 202–3.

which is imagined as male. When the female body is imagined, it is with reference to this male norm, so that there is an implicit hierarchy in play. Female bodies are male bodies with a difference. That is why the Galenic physician of *Medical Definitions* asks whether women are the same as men, and not the more open question of whether men and women are the same. The male, in other words, is the norm. Where female physiology and male physiology differ, male physiology is the norm from which the female diverges.[24] This philosophico-medical preference for the male body continued into modernity. Leonardo da Vinci's famous drawing, *Vitruvian Man*, an idealized naked body in two superimposed postures, designed so as to fit within a circle and square, is necessarily male precisely because it is intended to represent an ideal.

At the beginning of this chapter, and with the same subtle bias, we wondered why women seem twice as likely to suffer from depression as men. Would this 'fact' have looked as surprising if instead we had said that men are half as likely to suffer from depression as women? Might this second way of presenting the 'fact' have led to a different line of investigation? Instead of asking what makes women apparently more prone to depression, we might have asked what appears to give men greater immunity from depression. (One candidate: traditional male social roles such as hunting, soldiering, lawmaking, and priesthood do not require or reward much emotional engagement.) That is to say, how is our perspective affected by the decision to treat men as the norm and women as somehow aberrant? This may not be as explicit as the sexism of Aristotle, but it is responsible for insidious and pervasive gender bias nonetheless.

Our culture abounds in opposed pairs of concepts. While apparently of equal status ('man', 'woman'), many of them are in fact subtly asymmetrical – a phenomenon known as 'markedness' that was first observed in linguistics. In a given pair of terms the unmarked one is the universal or dominant term ('male', 'man'), and the marked term is the inflected, derived, or secondary one ('*f*emale', '*wo*man'). Applying the idea of markedness to culture in general exposes deep structural biases in the way we think.[25] Aristotle cites a list of opposed pairs apparently originating from Pythagorean philosophy. The list is headed by the cardinal pair 'male/female', and includes other pairs such as 'straight/curved', 'light/darkness', and 'good/evil'.[26] Aristotle gives no rationale for aligning *male*

---

[24] *Ibid.*, 89, 207–9.
[25] See Linda Waugh, 'Marked and Unmarked: A Choice Between Unequals in Semiotic Structure', *Semiotica* 38 (1982), 299–318.
[26] Ian Maclean, *The Renaissance Notion of Woman: A Study in the Fortunes of Scholasticism and Medical Science in European Intellectual Life* (Cambridge University Press, 1980), 2–3.

with *straight*, *light*, and *good*, and against *female*, *curved*, *darkness*, and *evil*, but it does not take much imagination or an overly cynical mind to come up with an explanation. *Male* and its allies are the unmarked terms: universal and dominant. *Female* and its allies are marked, derivative, secondary, and quite clearly deficient.

To summarize, gender bias has various sources, and the gendering of a complex concept like melancholia can take a number of different forms. Sometimes the forms of gendering combine, resulting in complex effects. Sometimes effects that operate elsewhere in culture seem not to affect melancholia at all or vice versa. Deep structures such as marked dualisms can affect nearly all aspects of a culture. Still, we need to be cautious about the sort of culturally totalizing argument that claims that *all the way down* culture is gendered in a manner unfavourable to women. It has frequently been observed that representations of melancholia as an embodied person in literature and art are traditionally female, whether the figure of 'Dame Merencolie' in Alain Chartier's early fifteenth-century lyrics or Albrecht Dürer's famous 1514 engraving *Melencolia I* or Lukas Cranach the Elder's allegorical painting *Melancholy* (1532). Whether this says anything significant about the gendering of melancholia is a moot point. Western culture has traditionally made personified abstractions female, whether negative (Melancholia) or positive (Justice). So it is hard to see the female gendering of personified abstractions either as specific to melancholia or as an effect of markedness in general. Less general and more helpful for our purposes is the gendering of the underlying physiological models used by Aristotle and the Graeco-Roman physicians (or some of them). In this case it is clear how the gendering of the medical theory directly determines the structure of the disease concept melancholia, so as to make women more prone to suffering from it or liable to experience it in specifically female ways. The link between physiology in general and specific disease concepts is especially strong in the rationalistic form of medical theory espoused by Galen and his followers. But we still need to be alert to the possibility that an individual physician might resist the implications of the physiological theory and produce an idiosyncratic version of melancholia that is gendered differently or for different reasons. In other words, arguments for the socio-historical or logical necessity of a particular form of gendering need to be tempered by sensitivity to human contingency. On a still smaller scale, the contact between melancholia and other, related concepts can produce gendering effects when the gendering of one concept infects another – what one might term gendering by contamination. And in cases like this, one would have to trace where the gendering comes from. Far less commonly, it seems, conceptions of melancholia are structured in such a way as to produce gender bias quite independently of their general cultural or medical context. This may result from the way in which melancholia and related concepts have been cut up, so as to include or exclude certain gender-specific phenomena such as female reproductive biology. A further possibility is that gender-neutral concepts might be applied in a gender-biased fashion by an overwhelmingly male medical profession.

4   Melancholia in the Christian Middle Ages

We have seen how some of the physiological models developed in Graeco-Roman medicine generated explicit and implicit gender bias. The subsequent history of melancholia also shows gendering at work in its full diversity and complexity. The Western Judaeo-Christian tradition largely accepted Aristotle's image of imperfect woman. Judaeo-Christian religion also added its own deep structural gender biases, of morality, psychology, and physiology. The lot of woman, according to Genesis 3:16, is sorrow, the pains of childbirth, and subordination to man. (Christian writers might have concluded from this malediction that women are more prone to melancholia than men, but they appear not to have done so.) Jewish law stigmatizes menstruation as unclean. In Leviticus the Lord commands segregation of menstruating women, along with much bathing or laundering of anyone or anything that has come into contact with them.[27] Medieval writers would explain menses in terms of the malediction on woman in Genesis. (Some non-medical writers in antiquity had also stressed the malignity of menstruation, but the ancient medical writers had specific medical reasons for taking a more positive view, as we will see.)[28]

A generally negative view of woman, in accord with Aristotle, could, of course, be justified by Christian theology. The sin of Eve betrayed the special weakness of the female flesh and spirit. Against this many writers, increasingly during the Renaissance, felt the need to defend the honour of woman. A stock discussion concerned the moral merit or otherwise of woman. Was woman 'bad woman' (*mala mulier*) or 'good woman' (*bona mulier*)? Of course, the very possibility of such a debate suggests the underlying markedness of *woman*. Some writers evidently felt the need to define woman by an additional moral qualification that was not felt necessary in the case of man.

How are the underlying biases of Judaeo-Christian thought reflected in medieval writers on melancholia? Most medical and philosophical writers

---

[27] For instance, Leviticus 15:19–30, 20:18; Ezekiel 18:5–6.
[28] Maclean, *Renaissance Notion*, 39.

followed the Aristotelian tradition as it had been mediated through medieval Islamic writers, and they reproduced its endemic prejudices. One interesting case is the twelfth-century German Benedictine abbess, mystic, composer, and polymath Hildegard von Bingen. The account of melancholia in her *Causes and Cures* is interesting not least because it is the earliest account of melancholia by a woman (assuming that she was indeed the author of *Causes and Cures*).[29] Also, Hildegard was philosophically and medically learned, and her learning presents a typical amalgam of Christian and classical arguments, the medicine being broadly classical, and the theology Christian. The underlying physiology is Aristotelian. Women are imperfect versions of men.[30] Woman's role in procreation is almost entirely passive and receptive, as envisaged by Aristotle. On the question of marriage, Hildegard suggests that melancholic women are better off without men, as men will tend to shun and mistreat them, knowing that the coldness of melancholy women makes them unlikely to bear children. Hildegard shows some sympathy towards melancholic women in their social exclusion, and she envisages one circumstance in which they might be received back into society. Exceptionally, a man of sanguine constitution can make a good husband for a melancholy woman, because of his natural warmth. By virtue of masculine warmth his sperm is hot enough to counteract the cooling effects of a melancholy wife, so ensuring that conception can occur, which is impossible with husbands of a cooler temperament.[31]

In either case, whether married to a sanguine man or following Hildegard's advice to remain safely chaste, the female melancholic, like woman in general, is marked as inferior to man and a prisoner of her reproductive physiology.[32] The primary feature of female melancholics is that they are normally incapable of procreation. Hildegard is by no means unusual in connecting melancholia with sex. There is a long tradition of viewing sexual dysfunction as key to the causes of and cures for melancholia. Sexual intercourse was recommended as a cure for melancholia by Rufus, though he probably only had male patients in mind. The Persian medical writer ar-Rāzī advises that men suffering from melancholia will improve their mood by having intercourse with slave girls.[33] Hildegard's argument comes instead from the misogynist Aristotle. Its presupposition would seem to be that marriage is the only way for a woman to overcome

---

[29] On doubts about attribution, see Margret Berger's preface to Hildegard of Bingen, *On Natural Philosophy and Medicine*, ed. and trans. Margret Berger (Cambridge: Brewer, 1999), ix–xv (at pp. x–xi).
[30] Schiesari, *Gendering*, 151.   [31] *Ibid.*, 152.   [32] *Ibid.*, 153.
[33] Peter E. Pormann and Emilie Savage-Smith, *Medieval Islamic Medicine* (Edinburgh University Press, 2007), 49.

her innate physiological and psychological lack and so become perfect like a man.[34] This belief has enjoyed a long history. In the late eighteenth century Hoffmann argued that 'of madness in young women from love, the most effectual remedy is marriage'.[35]

Hildegard also has an unmarked, non-gynaecological version of melancholia, though in an indirect way it is also connected with sexual physiology. Like all things human, melancholia derives its character from the seed of Adam. Hildegard here produces a version of Graeco-Roman humoral theory adapted to Old Testament theology:

> *Melancholic persons.* There are persons who are sad and fearful and vacillate in their moods so that there exists no right disposition and state for them. They are like a strong wind that is useless for all plants and fruit. From this a *flegma* grows in them that is neither moist nor dense but tepid … It produces black bile that first originated from Adam's semen through the breath of the serpent, since Adam heeded its counsel in taking food.[36]

Hildegard might have chosen to locate the cause of melancholia in the weakness of Eve or the malediction of woman in Leviticus. By instead choosing Adam as the source of melancholia, she cleaves to Aristotle's view of the physiological nature of melancholia, in the sense that all human physiology is ultimately determined by the condition of the male seed. As we have seen, in Aristotelian biology it is the male seed that determines reproduction, not the female womb (except insofar as the womb hinders full expression of the seed). So the choice of Adam as the father of melancholia conforms to the common Aristotelian prejudice against women, *pace* attempts by recent feminist critics to cast Hildegard as a proto-feminist.[37] Nor is there any evidence of a specifically male gendering of melancholia. Adam's seed may be the source of melancholia, but the melancholia it generates affects men and women equally.

With the epidemic growth of belief in witchcraft and demonic possession in early modern Europe, another distinctively Christian form of melancholia emerged. Here a number of factors combined to produce strong gendering effects. The practice of magic was part of the ancient European folk tradition, but there is no evidence that magic and melancholia were connected in the Graeco-Roman sources, except insofar as Rufus of Ephesus credited melancholics with the ability to predict the future.[38] The contact between witchcraft and melancholia was very much a product of the early modern period. Early modern witchcraft was, of course, highly gendered. Women outnumbered men as defendants in

[34] Maclean, *Renaissance Notion*, 8.   [35] Hoffmann, *System*, 298–303.
[36] Hildegard, *On Natural Philosophy*, 27.   [37] Schiesari, *Gendering*, 145–59.
[38] Rufus, *On Melancholy*, 47.

witch trials by as many as twenty to one.[39] This may have been because women were the most dependent members of society and therefore the more easily accused and convicted.[40] The gendering of witchcraft also played to easy traditional prejudices about women. Witches were infamous for their promiscuity and were believed to indulge in sexual congress with the devil. This image of lustful woman cohered with the weakness of the flesh that Eve had bequeathed to all women. As Burton asked, 'Of women's unnaturall, unsatiable lust, what country, what Village doth not complaine?'[41]

A woman's physiology was believed to put her at acute risk of demonic possession. The risk was thought to be especially high for post-menopausal women, not least because of their natural dryness and susceptibility to melancholia.[42] The dryness of post-menopausal women was derived from traditional views about the function of the womb. Once women ceased to be reproductively active, their wombs, no longer lubricated by semen, wandered the body in search of lubrication. The result was hysteria, the disease of the wandering womb. It could afflict any woman who was not sexually active, hence Burton's chapter on 'Maides, Nunnes, and Widowes Melancholy'.[43]

Witches, being female, were more liable to suffer from melancholy vapours.[44] Ironically, this very gendering of melancholia would provide ammunition for rationalists who were sceptical about the whole theory of demonic possession. Did these so-called witches really practise demonic magic? Since women were known to be prone to melancholia, might not the practice of witchcraft in fact be a product of women's melancholy delusions? The Dutch physician Jan Wier (1515–1588) argued that a true pact with the devil was impossible. Any woman who claimed to have made one was merely suffering from melancholic delusions.[45] Oddly, this did not prevent Wier from believing that women were subject to demonic influence. In fact, he thought that a pre-existing psychic or physical propensity to melancholia could be exploited by the devil to lead the poor melancholic woman astray.[46] It was one of those strange arguments that only a period of religious extremism could produce, but by the

[39] Keith Thomas, *Religion and the Decline of Magic* (Harmondsworth: Penguin, 1971), 620.
[40] *Ibid.*, 678.   [41] Burton, *Anatomy*, vol. III, 55.
[42] Midelfort, *A History of Madness*, 69.   [43] Burton, *Anatomy*, vol. I, 414–18.
[44] Jackson, *Melancholia*, 329.   [45] Midelfort, *Madness*, 209.
[46] Annemarie Leibbrand-Wettley, 'Zur Psychopathologie und Dämonoligie bei Paracelsus und Johannes Weyer', in Joseph Schumacher, unter Mitarbeit von Martin Schrenk and Jörn Henning Wolf (eds.), *Melemata: Festschrift für Werner Leibbrand zum siebzigsten Geburtstag* (Mannheimer Großdruckerei, 1967), 65–73.

seventeenth century Wier's argument was deemed sufficiently strong to be used in courts of law, an early form of the insanity plea. Melancholia thus entered the canon of forensic literature.[47] In 1635 the German jurist Benedikt Carpzov was able to argue successfully for leniency in the punishment of melancholics.[48] Women were victims of their physiological and hence also psychological weakness; they were not witches in league with Satan.

5   Melancholy genius in early modern Europe

If the history of the gendering of melancholia tells one consistent story, it is that female melancholia is part of a general presumption of female divergence from a universal norm of male rationality. Feminist critics and historians have rightly stressed that the potential for this type of gendering was dramatically heightened when the idea of melancholy genius came into fashion in the Renaissance. The pseudo-Aristotelian *Problems* XXX/1 had been translated into Latin as early as the thirteenth century, but it had to wait until the late fifteenth century to be rediscovered by the Florentine Neoplatonist philosopher Marsilio Ficino. Normally attributed to Aristotle, the text was probably authored by Theophrastus (*c*. 371– *c*. 287 BC), Aristotle's successor as head of the Peripatetic school of philosophy. Despite its sound Aristotelian pedigree, the text contains some distinctly Platonic elements. These may have made it uncongenial to the dominant neo-Aristotelian philosophy of the late Middle Ages and may explain why little attention had been paid to it before Ficino. It begins by asking a striking question:

Why is it that all men who have become outstanding in philosophy, statesmanship, poetry or the arts are melancholic, and some to such an extent that they are infected by the diseases arising from black bile, as the story of Heracles among the heroes tells?[49]

A version of the argument connecting melancholia with brilliance appears in later Graeco-Roman medical theory; for instance, Rufus states that people 'of excellent nature' are prone to melancholia.[50] The Persian physician and philosopher ar-Rāzī echoes Rufus in his *Comprehensive Book*, and the Latin translation of ar-Rāzī is quoted by Burton: 'And those who are of subtle mind and great insight easily succumb to

---

[47] Midelfort, *Madness*, 218–19.   [48] *Ibid.*, 222.

[49] Aristotle, *Problems*, trans. W. H. Hett, Loeb Classical Library, 2 vols. (Cambridge, MA: Harvard University Press, 1936–7), vol. II, 155.

[50] Rufus, *On Melancholy*, 47.

melancholia.'[51] In Rufus' version of the genius theory the genial melancholic is grammatically male gendered, as the normal usage of Ancient Greek required. Otherwise the passage is not obviously gendered. The pseudo-Aristotelian text, on the other hand, is gendered in ways that are not necessitated by normal linguistic practice. The text uses the word 'man' (*anēr, andr-*) throughout, and the examples it gives from history and myth are of male figures. There is no reference to melancholy women, despite their being discussed frequently in the Graeco-Roman medical literature. The attributes of the melancholic listed in the text, passion, desire, talkativeness, and creativity, are thus confirmed as male. The text also connects them to male social roles: the statesman, the philosopher, and the poet. It is also noteworthy that the pseudo-Aristotelian text, with its extravagant opening, strong male gendering, and male examples from myth and history, had very little influence on the medical tradition. It is clear the text was not written by a physician, unlike the other ancient writings on melancholia we know about.[52] Thanks to its distance from the medical tradition, the pseudo-Aristotelian text, on its rediscovery in the Renaissance, could appear quite fresh and distinct. Although of Aristotelian provenance, it was unencumbered by the philosophical baggage of neo-Aristotelian scholasticism and could therefore appeal to philosophers like Ficino who wanted to break with scholasticism and embrace Neoplatonist alternatives. It created a new norm of genial male melancholia that was philosophical and universal.

Shakespeare's Prince Hamlet has often been interpreted as a representative of this Neoplatonist Renaissance melancholia. Like the male melancholics of the pseudo-Aristotelian *Problems*, he possesses a rare gift for verbal virtuosity and a penchant for speculative reasoning. However, this interpretation is not without its difficulties. Aside from the understandable grief Hamlet feels for his father's death, some elements of Hamlet's melancholia appear to be 'put ... on' (Act I, scene v, line 170).[53] Nor is it by any means the pure genial melancholia. The piteous state in which he accosts Ophelia in her closet, by her report, offers a checklist of symptoms of early modern love melancholia:

> with his doublet all unbraced,
> No hat upon his head, his stockings fouled,
> Ungartered, and down-gyved to his ankle,

---

[51] Burton, *Anatomy*, vol. I, 165: the Latin is quoted in the footnote: 'qui sunt subtilis ingenii, & multae perspicacitatis de facili incidunt in Melancholiam'.

[52] Jouanna, 'At the Roots of Melancholy', 237–41.

[53] William Shakespeare, *Hamlet*, ed. Ann Thompson and Neil Taylor, The Arden Shakespeare (London: Thomson, 2006), 225.

> Pale as his shirt, his knees knocking each other,
> And with a look so piteous in purport
> As if he had been loosed out of hell
> To speak of horrors. . .
>
> (Act II, scene i, lines 75–81)[54]

This is a quite different tradition from the strong male genial melancholia of the *Problems*. Notwithstanding this difficulty, feminist critics have pointed to a strong gender contrast between Hamlet's melancholia and Ophelia's. She is presented as a classic case of female love melancholia, a 'document in madness', according to her brother Laertes. Her melancholia is marked as female by its specific focus on love in supposed contrast to Hamlet's more universal and metaphysical distress.[55] But the case of Ophelia is also complex. The sane Ophelia is a largely accepting and passive character, one who observes but does not intervene (Act III, scene i, line 160).[56] This is in the first place shown to be a product of social norms, in particular the subordination of women to men. Ophelia is governed by her father, her brother, and Hamlet. Even when mad, she shows no aggression or violence. Her 'plangent and gentle' madness is therefore best seen as an extension of her passive sane self,[57] only now she is disordered and distracted (Act IV, scene v, line 2).[58] It is a madness occupied with picking and braiding flowers and singing songs. The songs comment on her father Polonius's death and her loss of Hamlet's affection in an almost childish way, though they do briefly allude in faintly bawdy terms to an imagined sexual transgression (Act IV, scene v, lines 58–66)[59] – this is the chief plank of Elaine Showalter's argument that Ophelia is a classic erotomaniac. But the songs have nothing of the barely concealed obscenity and murderousness of the mad Gretchen's songs in Goethe's *Faust*, a character owing much to Ophelia, but altogether more active and sceptical and the perfect foil to Faust's truly genial melancholia. Their fates distinguish them clearly: Ophelia dies after she accidentally falls into a brook, to which she reacts with passive indifference, 'like a creature native and endued / Unto that element' (Act IV, scene vii, lines 177–8).[60] Gretchen in her madness murders her own child, as a reaction to having loved and lost Faust and, in the process, killed her mother and lost her brother. Finally she chooses not to let Faust rescue her from imminent execution, preferring instead to submit herself by her own

---

[54] *Ibid.*, 234.
[55] Elaine Showalter, *The Female Malady: Women, Madness, and English Culture, 1830–1980* (London: Virago, 1987), 11.
[56] Shakespeare, *Hamlet*, 293.
[57] Anne Barton, 'Introduction', in William Shakespeare, *Hamlet*, The New Penguin Shakespeare, ed. T. J. B. Spencer (London: Penguin, 1980), 7–54 (at p. 26).
[58] *Ibid.*, 372.   [59] *Ibid.*, 378.   [60] *Ibid.*, 408.

active volition to the mercy of God and the justice of the death sentence that has been passed on her. In both Ophelia and Gretchen, love melancholia is an extension of the original sane character. In neither case is the gendering a result of melancholia; on the contrary, their melancholia merely reflects a pre-existing socially determined gendering. Melancholia adds practically no effects of gendering to those found in society at large.

Even if the argument for the gendering of melancholia in *Hamlet* can only be accepted with reservations, it does show us a general truth about women's melancholia in the early modern period: the tendency to mark women's melancholia as love melancholia and so to diminish its status. It does not help that there are relatively few literary self-portrayals by melancholic women before the late seventeenth century.[61] This changed with the spread of Calvinist religious melancholia in the seventeenth century and the coming of the age of sensibility in the second quarter of the eighteenth. Numerous melancholy poems by women date from this period, and the evidence suggests that women did not indulge in Hamletesque philosophical melancholia.[62] Instead in this poetry women tend to expire through loneliness and the shame of being abandoned by their lovers.[63]

Better evidence for the gendering of melancholia than *Hamlet* is furnished by Goethe's great tragic novel of sensibility *The Sorrows of Young Werther*. The bourgeois anti-hero Werther runs the full gamut of melancholic types.[64] One is love melancholia; another is the philosophical male melancholic role – for instance, when he ruminates on the incapacity of human thought to capture the ineffable richness of nature. The Ophelia role falls to Werther's unavailable beloved Lotte. Of course, the feminized literary culture of sensibility causes a certain blurring of gender roles, since the man often takes on female characteristics. Werther suffers from love melancholia – or does he put it on like Hamlet? But while Werther is allowed to perform his melancholia in a number of frankly quite stagey ways, Lotte has (or desires) no such opportunity. She is something of a repressed melancholic. Only when Werther commits suicide does she reach a crisis, of which all we are told is that she fainted and 'there were fears for Lotte's life'.[65]

---

[61] Roy Porter, *A Social History of Madness: Stories of the Insane* (New York: Weidenfeld, 1987), 104.
[62] Eleanor Maria Sickels, *The Gloomy Egoist: Moods and Themes of Melancholy from Gray to Keats*. Columbia University Studies in English and Comparative Literature (New York: Columbia University Press, 1932), 204.
[63] *Ibid.*, 233–4.
[64] Thorsten Valk, *Melancholie im Werk Goethes* (Tübingen: Niemeyer, 2002), 69–77.
[65] Johann Wolfgang von Goethe, *The Sorrows of Young Werther*, trans. Michael Hulse (Harmondsworth: Penguin, 1989), 134.

6   Love melancholia

Hamlet and Werther notwithstanding, to what extent was love melancholia associated specifically with women? Love melancholia or *amor hereos* was a central feature of the culture of courtly love in the late Middle Ages, above all in Italian and French poetry. (The etymology of *hereos* is obscure, but its probably spurious associations with the idea of the heroic no doubt made it attractive, in contrast to common-or-garden melancholia.)[66] Traditional Christian teaching presented women as sinful and fleshly, and consequently more susceptible to love melancholia than men. However, in the 'heroic' tradition of lovesickness, men were at least as susceptible and, judging by Ophelia's readiness to decipher Hamlet's sloppy appearance, it was evidently a game that could be played by both sexes.

Quite how the symptoms of love melancholia related to underlying physiological models was also obscure. In his 1610 treatise on lovesickness the French physician Jacques Ferrand acknowledged that, according to medical theory, men should be more prone to love melancholia than women, because their physiology made them dryer.[67] Now, though, a broader and deeper prejudice kicks in. As love is opposed to reason, women, being less rational than men, should in theory experience more love melancholia than men. And so it proves in our daily experience, says Ferrand: we see more 'witless, maniacal and frantic' women than men. However, Ferrand is enough of a Galenic physician not to want to relinquish the idea that observation conforms to theory and observed behaviour is determined by physiology. The clinching physiological fact is that in men there is a greater distance between the sexual organs and the stomach, and this suggests that men, not by dint of any rational superiority but through brute physiology, are capable of greater temperance than women, simply because their spermatic vessels are less liable to be heated by the stomach than a woman's womb is.[68] Here Ferrand reproduces a traditional Graeco-Roman focus on the sperm as the defining feature of a gendered physiology. From the Renaissance onwards, love melancholia would be closely implicated in theories about male and female reproductive physiology.

The decisive feature of female reproductive physiology was the womb. Whereas the Old Testament had stigmatized menstruation, Graeco-

---

[66] Roger Boase, *The Origin and Meaning of Courtly Love: A Critical Study of European Scholarship* (Manchester University Press, 1977), 132–3.

[67] Jacques Ferrand, *A Treatise on Lovesickness*, trans. and ed. by Donald A. Beecher and Massimo Ciavolella (Syracuse, NY: Syracuse University Press, 1990), 311.

[68] *Ibid.*, 312.

Roman medicine presented a more nuanced, though still biased, picture of menstruation. Much Graeco-Roman therapy was concerned with the purging of the blood in order to purify it of unhealthy elements. Female menstruation, a natural and regular form of bloodletting, was therefore of obvious interest to medical writers. Graeco-Roman physicians stressed that full and proper menstruation is vital to a woman's health. Like Hippocrates before him, Galen held that full menstruation confers immunity from disease. He wrote that a 'well-purged woman' is immune to a whole range of diseases, including melancholia.[69] By 'well-purged', Galen implies that a woman's menses vary from month to month in their quantity and quality. (Graeco-Roman physicians seem to have been more interested in the quantity and quality of the menses than their timing, which may be of more urgent concern to women themselves.) In some months the menstrual flow is more copious and therefore healthier than in others. So while at first sight it might appear that menstrual immunity from disease gives women an inbuilt health advantage over men, on closer inspection we see that women are subject to more variability and instability in their health from month to month than men, and this might further be interpreted as confirmation of the Aristotelian prejudice against women. This general concern about women's health appears not to have led to the conclusion that women are more likely to suffer from melancholia. While Graeco-Roman physicians did blame the womb for all manner of illnesses, they did not identify the womb as a location of the noxious melancholic humour.[70] By the sixteenth century, however, this had changed. Burton wrote that melancholia could be caused by the 'vicious vapours that come from menstruous blood', especially when the blood was not properly evacuated through menstruation. This was one reason why melancholia could be more acute in spinsters, nuns, widows, and pregnant women, '*ob suppressam purgationem*' – because the purification of the blood in menstruation had been suppressed.[71] From Galen to Burton the relation between melancholia and menstruation had turned through 180 degrees.

7   Gender in early modern medicine

In the late seventeenth century, physicians went one step further and drew a connection between melancholia hypochondriaca and the classically female disease of hysteria. Hysteria was by definition female; originally it

---

[69] Flemming, *Medicine*, 338.
[70] Andrew T. Scull, *Hysteria: The Biography* (Oxford University Press, 2009), 13.
[71] Burton, *Anatomy*, vol. I, 414.

merely designated a medical condition of the womb and did not necessarily involve psychological symptoms. This changed when seventeenth-century physicians linked hysteria to melancholia hypochondriaca and created a specifically female mental disorder. By way of a complement to hysterical hypochondria, the physicians also constructed a specifically male form of melancholia or hypochondria, drawing on the ancient connection of melancholia with epilepsy. For instance, George Cheyne (1671–1743) tends to describe male hypochondria as 'Epileptick' and female as 'Hysterick'.[72] A further connection could then be made to the pseudo-Aristotelian and Renaissance notions of melancholy genius. With Cheyne, hypochondriasis became the disease of the (male) genius. This modern genial hypochondriasis took on the colours of its century. Unlike the solitary melancholy geniuses of the Renaissance, Cheyne's eighteenth-century hypochondriac geniuses were sociable, sharing in what Cheyne saw as the benefits and ills of the century's intense sociability.[73] So hysteria was incorporated into melancholia, and brought with it the gendering that was hysteria's birthright[74] – a classic case of gendering by contamination, but also characteristic of a more general tendency towards gender differentiation in mental illness that set in in the late eighteenth century.[75]

At the dawn of the modern period, physicians faced both forwards and backwards. Innovation came in the form of new discoveries in empirical anatomy, by such giants of Renaissance medicine as Andreas Vesalius (1514–1564). But as we saw in Chapter 1, Renaissance medicine was also inspired by the new humanist editions of Hippocrates and Galen. The aim was to return to the pure ancient sources and cleanse them of all the distortions, confusions, and accretions of over a thousand years of tradition. Physicians questioned the authority of Aristotle, who was in any case a philosopher and not a physician, and was considered by some to be a vulgar plagiarist of Hippocrates.[76] Some 'feminist' physicians even objected to the Philosopher's misogynist physiological theory, and after 1600 most physicians seem to have rejected the Aristotelian view of sex difference. However, continuing adherence to Hippocrates and Galen meant that the new Renaissance medicine could not escape other, less acute forms of gendering. Indeed, the shift in physiological thinking that began in the seventeenth century brought with it new possibilities for the

---

[72] G. J. Barker-Benfield, *The Culture of Sensibility: Sex and Society in Eighteenth-Century Britain* (University of Chicago Press, 1992), 25; Jackson, *Melancholia*, 139.

[73] Roy Porter, 'Introduction', in George Cheyne, *The English Malady* (London: Routledge, 1991), xxxviii.

[74] Scull, *Hysteria*, 35.   [75] Showalter, *Female Malady*, 8.

[76] Maclean, *Renaissance Notion*, 28.

gendering of melancholia, as we have already seen in the case of hysterical hypochondria. The move towards a nerve-based theory of physiology – for instance, in the work of Thomas Willis (1621–1675) – became particularly important not only in medicine but also in European culture more widely after 1700. The implications of nervous theory for the gendering of melancholia were twofold. Their refined and delicate nerves made women more susceptible to disease.[77] (Aristotle, still refusing to die, had determined that women's bodies and minds were softer.) Women were therefore more susceptible to external influences and so more liable to be made melancholy by shocks and upsets such as lost love (though Burton had listed many such afflictions as causes of women's melancholia).[78] On the other hand, the rise of the new culture of sensibility from around 1720 gave new, positive value to women's receptivity, for better or worse. The renewed vogue for melancholia in the literature of the mid 1700s contributed to the feminization of literary culture, as we have already noted, though, as often as not, the positive values associated with women were constructions foisted on them by men. And even when women were credited with sensibility, they could still be denied (male) intelligence and genius. As the German medical writer Ernst Platner noted in 1776, women have 'a soft and dull brain, albeit one occasionally sensitive to physical pain'.[79]

After 1800 the link between melancholia and genius was gradually severed. With melancholia no longer defined in terms of male genius, a more decisive move towards the female gendering of melancholia (and eventually depression) could begin. Melancholia could become the disease of nervous women. In 1845 Thomas Laycock observed that women were more highly strung and 'more liable to all diseases of excitement'.[80] There was indeed a perception that women were more prone to mental illness in general, and a myth developed that the asylums of Europe were filling with women – a myth not borne out by the statistics of asylum admissions. What is certainly true is that more women than men were being treated by private 'nerve doctors' for nervous disorders such as melancholia and asthenia,[81] a tendency reflected in the classic nineteenth-century picture of the neurasthenic woman confined to bed for a 'rest cure'.[82] Melancholic men, of course,

---

[77] Barker-Benfield, *Culture of Sensibility*, 345.
[78] Bell, *The German Tradition of Psychology*, ch. 3.
[79] Ernst Platner, *Philosophische Aphorismen, nebst einigen Anleitungen zur philosophischen Geschichte*, 2 vols. (Leipzig: Schwickert, 1776–82), vol. I, 286.
[80] Lisa Appignanesi, *Mad, Bad and Sad: A History of Women and the Mind Doctors from 1800* (London: Virago, 2009), 119.
[81] *Ibid.*, 107.   [82] Radden, *Nature of Melancholy*, 18.

had traditionally been prescribed the opposite, the 'activity cure': Werther's mother and his correspondent Wilhelm see activity as the cure for his melancholia.

8   Continuity and complexity

One noteworthy feature of the gendering of modern depression is its continuity with trends that began in much earlier periods. The nineteenth-century image of the passive depressed woman continues an older Aristotelian view of woman as passive (not least in matters of reproduction). One could make a similar point concerning the tendency to connect melancholia with reproductive physiology, which began in the Middle Ages (see Hildegard), increased in prominence in the early modern period (Ferrand's theory of love melancholia), and continues today in DSM-5's categorization of premenstrual tension as a form of depressive disorder. Perhaps this should not surprise us: the dismantling of millennia of cultural gendering is not likely to happen overnight. What these continuities reveal above all is that for hundreds of years medical theory has combined with much broader forms of traditional misogyny to produce gendered physiological models. Melancholia is no more and no less than part of the highly gendered picture of Western medicine in general.

Equally, it is unfair to blame everything on Aristotle, tempting though it may be. The question of the gendering of melancholia is complex. Often the primary vehicles of gendering were neighbouring non-medical concepts (such as genius or sensibility) or underlying belief systems (such as the Judaeo-Christian belief in the sinfulness of the flesh). And the reasons for the gendering of medical theories are by no means all to be ascribed to the Philosopher. For one thing, most ancient physicians were not Aristotelians, and many modern physicians explicitly rejected Aristotle's influence. In some periods and in some medical theories the construction of melancholia does seem to have had its own gendering that was particular to the institution of medicine and had nothing to do with Aristotle. This may have been because of the way disease categories were cut up, or because the focus of physicians was drawn to particular phenomena. We also should not discount the possibility that gender-neutral concepts were applied in biased ways. There is ample reason to be suspicious of a medical profession which until the twentieth century was almost exclusively male, and whose higher echelons are still pre-dominantly male in most parts of the world. Recent feminist research on the history of mental illness has focused on the way in which 'the essential feminine nature unveil[s] itself before scientific male rationality'.[83] Where men are the agents of medicine and women its objects, some bias is inevitable.

But totalizing arguments of this kind can be unhelpful. Although melancholia shows a remarkable empirical consistency, the theoretical models that purport to account for melancholia – Jackson's 'parade of theories' – show great diversity across time and space, as we saw in Chapter 2. Because melancholia is made up of various elements that interlock in complex ways, we need to tread carefully when looking for gendering in melancholia. Sometimes an otherwise gender-neutral concept can be infected by gender biases in another related concept. And major differences exist between concepts of melancholia through history but also between different medical writers at the same time. We should not expect to find a clear or uniform picture.

The impression of a higher incidence of melancholia in one gender than the other may also be a product of biases in empirical observation. Even though physicians may be operating in good faith, empirical observation is not gender-neutral. Before the modern period, problems of small sample sizes and untested assumptions meant that, even in the case of a well-documented body of reports like Napier's, the evidence is unlikely to be methodologically robust. Even in contemporary medicine with its large sample sizes and carefully calibrated statistical approaches, gender biases, whether conscious or unconscious, can play a role. Biased categories will pick up biased results. This, as we have seen, applies today as much as it did in Ancient Greece. DSM-5, in use since 2013, is hardly gender-neutral.

---

[83] Showalter, *Female Malady*, 3.

4   The Western malady

1   From gender bias to cultural bias

Are women human beings? Flippant and obnoxious though the question might be, one can almost imagine it being asked by a medieval Aristotelian. (A similar question was in fact asked: 'is woman a monstrous creation?' The answer was almost always 'no'.)[1] The question might also be asked as a rhetorical foil by a modern feminist criticizing Aristotelian misogyny. The feminist would have a point. The same male-dominated science that marks female melancholia as divergent from unmarked male melancholia has traditionally insisted that a single disease entity *melancholia* is experienced in all cultures. If melancholia is the same for all humans except women, does this mean women are not human?

Perhaps any realist psychiatry risks falling into this trap. If sadness is a universal affect, as Ekman and others have argued, then melancholia and depression would also be strong contenders for universality. In one form or another this universalist view has been held by almost all psychiatrists, including those who have studied the cultural variability of mental disorders. This is despite the wide geographical variations in the incidence of symptoms of depression that research in cross-cultural psychiatry has revealed. A World Health Organization survey published in 1983 studied the symptoms of depression in a series of sample groups from different geographical locations worldwide. The survey showed that while patients shared a core of symptoms that were present in 76 to 100 per cent of each sample, there was wide variation between samples in the frequency of other symptoms. For instance, the Iranian sample showed a very high incidence of psychomotor agitation (e.g. repeated touching of the face, pacing around the room, wringing of hands). Feelings of guilt and self-reproach, on the other hand, were high in the Western European

---

[1] Maclean, *Renaissance Notion*, 30–1.

sample (68 per cent of patients) and much lower in Iran (32 per cent).[2] More striking differences have emerged from studies of depression in China, where the typical Western phenomena of depressed mood and anxiety seem to be largely absent. Depression in China presents much like nineteenth-century neurasthenia, with symptoms of fatigue, sleep disturbance, stomach pains, and hypertension.[3] This has led medical anthropologists, or at least Western medical anthropologists, to classify the Chinese form as 'masked depression', a form of depression that is prevented by Chinese cultural norms from reaching full psychological expression. The presumption is that there is a universal (non-masked, unmarked) form of depression – the normative Western form with all its florid psychological symptoms of anhedonia, self-loathing, guilt, pessimism, and so on – from which the (masked, marked) Chinese form diverges. In other words it looks as if the biases caused by gendering in medicine repeat themselves in cross-cultural studies of depression.

The source of this problem lies in a particular conception of *medical* psychiatry. There is an easy presumption that since medicine is concerned with biological processes, a medically oriented psychiatry must be chiefly concerned with biology. On this view, mental disorders are biological facts; depression is a symptom of faulty brain chemistry. If this were true, it would be natural to conclude that mental disorders are just as universal as physical illnesses. But as we saw in the Introduction, a medical psychiatry does not inevitably imply that mental disorders are universal.[4] The causes of mental disorders might just as well be social as physical. Mental disorders might therefore be specific to their sociocultural contexts. It will follow from this that Western depression is just as much a cultural construct as Chinese depression. There is nothing universal or unmarked about Western depression. Western psychiatrists might have set up Western depression as a universal norm from which marked Chinese depression supposedly diverges, but there are no rational grounds for doing so. Why should we privilege Western depression like this? Is this anything more than a Western cultural prejudice? Is it any different from the Western medical tradition's habit of marking female melancholia?

At the same time as guarding against universalism, we need to avoid parochialism. Some historians of early modern melancholia have been

---

[2] N. Sartorius *et al.*, *Depressive Disorders in Different Cultures: Report on the WHO Collaborative Study on Standardized Assessment of Depressive Disorders* (Geneva: World Health Organization, 1983), 92.

[3] Arthur Kleinman, *Social Origins of Distress and Disease: Depression, Neurasthenia and Pain in Modern China* (Newhaven, CT: Yale University Press, 1988), 52–5.

[4] Murphy, *Psychiatry in the Scientific Image*, 279–80.

persuaded by the claims, made by Burton and his contemporaries, that Europe was experiencing an epidemic of melancholia. This melancholia would thus appear to have been a product of early modern conditions. Historians have sought to explain the supposed early modern epidemic in terms of socio-cultural changes, most notably the rise of modern individualism. Melancholia, they contend, became endemic in the West when a specifically capitalist form of individualism emerged, beginning in Renaissance Italy. A similar argument has been made for our own period. The current epidemic of depression has its roots in the fragmenting of post-modern capitalist societies. The post-modern media alienate us from reality. Advertising stimulates inauthentic desires in us for a world we cannot possess. Spiritual solidarity is torn asunder by the modern world of work and its relentless march towards the division of labour. Social solidarity breaks down as turbo-capitalism increases the gulf between rich and poor. As plausible as these explanations may sound, they fail to account for large parts of melancholia's history, most obviously Graeco-Roman and medieval Islamic melancholia. In this sense it seems justified to call them parochial. There is nothing wrong with their logic; what is wrong is their narrow field of view. They fail to account for anything beyond the modern period, whereas the phenomenon they purport to explain extends back to the fifth century BC.

This chapter addresses the geographical and historical variability of melancholia. Its premise is that in their different ways geography and history create the conditions for the existence of culture-bound syndromes. The niche in which a syndrome emerges and flourishes is bounded by historical time and geographical space. More specifically, it is bounded by particular cultural forms: Graeco-Roman medicine and the cultures of self-consciousness that have existed in the West since antiquity.

2   The cultural anthropology of mental disorders

The West has tended to apply different standards to its own and to non-Western mental disorders, despite the evident irrationality of doing so. This is not to impute any sinister intent to Western psychiatrists or anthropologists of psychiatry. The double standard is more the result of underlying cultural biases and the ways these have caused disciplinary boundaries to be drawn, such as the boundary between psychiatry and anthropology. While Western mental disorders have been the disciplinary province of a biologically oriented and universalizing psychiatry, non-Western mental disorders were the province of a culturally oriented and particularizing anthropology. In the view of Western psychiatry, Western mental disorders were as real and universal as influenza; they were to be defined and treated by a medical science of psychiatry. Non-Western disorders were forms of culturally specific behaviour; their governing science was anthropology. Or to put it another way, the realist position that I staked out in this book's Introduction requires that a medically oriented psychiatry be the proper discipline for mental disorders, whether Western or not, but that all psychiatry is also culturally constructed, whether the disorders it studies are at home or abroad.

There is nothing wrong in principle with an anthropology of mental disorders, but it does carry risks. One risk is the possibility of contamination by Western imperialist and racist ideologies, with their tendency to treat non-Western peoples as racially or culturally inferior. A recurrent theme in the anthropology of mental disorders is the failure of non-Western cultures to experience anything as rich as Western depression. Instead of suffering from the complex and florid psychological symptoms of true depression, non-Westerners experience an impoverished form of depression that presents as mere bodily malaise. J. C. Carothers, writing about depression in Africa in the 1950s, explained the absence of psychological symptoms and presence instead of bodily symptoms in terms of the cultural backwardness of the indigenous peoples: '[T]he African with his slight ability for introspection and for discrimination between body and mind, would tend to identify a feeling of depression with bodily ill-health.'[5] The literature on Chinese masked depression is much less obviously prejudiced, but it still contains an implicit bias. Chinese masked depression presents as a set of physiological symptoms, without the strong feelings of loss and sadness that characterize Western depression. The absence of Western psychological symptoms is explained in terms of Chinese culture's inhibitions. Chinese patients' '"feelings" are private and embarrassing events that are best not explored'. Psychological insight would mean potentially shameful 'self-absorption'.[6] This model improves on Carothers by explaining the differences in terms of cultural norms rather than cultural backwardness. But the underlying model of depression is still the Western psychological one: Chinese depression is seen as an incomplete form of full Western depression. By implication, non-Western illnesses are subaltern forms of Western ones.

[5] J. C. Carothers, 'Frontal Lobe Function and the African', *Journal of Mental Sciences* 97 (1951), 12–48.
[6] Catherine Lutz, 'Depression and the Translation of Emotional Worlds', in Arthur Kleinman and Byron Good (eds.), *Culture and Depression* (Berkeley, CA: University of California Press, 1985), 63–100 (at p. 70).

Some of these biases can be avoided if instead of applying Western nosological models, anthropologists focus on syndromes that are specific to non-Western cultures and are recognized as syndromes by the local medical practitioners. But here another risk emerges: the fascination of the Western anthropological gaze with the exotic and spectacular. A rich anthropological literature has grown up around these (mainly psychotic) non-Western syndromes. Most famous is the *amok* or *amuck* of Malaysia, Indonesia, and the Philippines. A state brought on by stress or grief and most often found among males, *amok* displays symptoms ranging from depression, confusion, and worry, to acute cases in which a self-induced trance evolves into a frenzy of violence.[7] Malaysian *latah* is another condition brought on by stress. Sufferers exhibit uncontrolled behaviour often involving imitation of another person's movement and speech, automatic obedience, and sexual delusions.[8] Among the Arctic Inuit, anthropologists have found the syndrome of 'kayak fright': dizziness, palpitations, sweating, and paralysis accompany the understandably alarming delusion that one's kayak is filling with water.[9] A syndrome experienced in the Spanish-speaking Caribbean, *ataques de nervios*, involves 'a sudden, though transient, change in behaviour that occurs after a major stress'. Symptoms include 'changes in the level of consciousness and amnesia ... sudden or impulsive behaviour such as suicide attempts, falling to the floor, assaultiveness and seizure-like activity'.[10] The 'windigo psychosis' found among young males of the Ojibwa, Algonquin, and Cree nations of North America is a deep depression involving delusions and occasional cannibalism.[11] Last but not least in our tour of worldwide mental illness, the Pokot people of East Africa suffer from *kipoiyin* or a 'severe loss of sense'. A notable symptom is arson: 'a psychotic Pokot is very likely to set fire to a house, sometimes when the occupants are asleep inside'.[12]

---

[7] Eduardo Ugarte, 'The Demoniacal Impulse: The Construction of Amok in the Philippines', unpublished dissertation (University of Western Sydney, 1999).

[8] Robert L. Winzeler, *Latah in South-East Asia: The History and Ethnography of a Culture-Bound Syndrome* (Cambridge University Press, 1995).

[9] Seymour Parker, 'Eskimo Psychopathology in the Context of Eskimo Personality and Culture', *American Anthropologist* 64 (1962), 76–96.

[10] Maria Oquendo, Ewald Horwath, and Abigail Martinez, 'Ataques de Nervios: Proposed Diagnostic Criteria for a Culture-Specific Syndrome', *Culture, Medicine and Psychiatry* 16 (1992), 367–76 (at p. 368).

[11] Jeffrey Scott Mio et al. (eds.), *Key Words in Multicultural Interventions: A Dictionary* (Westport, CT; London: Greenwood, 1999), 269.

[12] Robert B. Edgerton, 'Conceptions of Psychosis in East-African Societies', in David Landy (ed.), *Culture, Disease, and Healing: Studies in Medical Anthropology* (New York: Macmillan, 1977), 358–67.

The purpose of this tour of mental disorders is decidedly not to denigrate them or to deny their reality. The question is not whether the syndromes are real. They are evidently real enough to the people who experience them. The point at issue is their appropriation and use by Western anthropology. The syndromes are of obvious interest to anthropologists, and therein lies the danger. They are what we might call 'spectaculars', the exotic objects of the fascinated Western anthropological gaze. The danger is that anthropologists can portray these spectacular psychoses as representative of their cultures as a whole, so that the cultures in turn appear exotic and unstable. Malay culture is somehow construed as a culture that generates *latah* and is thus marked as potentially undisciplined and given to sexual licence. In other words, there is a risk that this kind of anthropology turns foreign cultures into exotica and museum pieces that contrast with the norm of Western rationality.

The flaw in the search for analogues of depression is the implied presumption that Western depression, and specifically its culture-dependent psychological symptoms, should serve as some kind of norm. Where a syndrome is found that might serve as a potential analogue of Western depression, its deviance from Western depression comes to stand for the culture that produced it. The logic is correct, but what is often missed in these studies is that the appearance of deviance is an artefact of perspective. These spectacular syndromes seem deviant to us only because we think of our own Western culture as unmarked and gifted with a universal scientific rationality.

By shifting our perspective it is possible to see things differently, and some cross-cultural psychiatrists have done this successfully. A study published in 2008 examined samples of depressed patients in the USA and China, and found that Chinese patients tended to refer to somatic symptoms, while US patients would present with more psychological symptoms. The study then turned traditional wisdom on its head. Instead of arguing that Chinese depression is somehow incomplete, it pointed out that the biological symptoms seemed to be universal and the psychological ones culturally specific. Depression begins with a biological response, and this gives rise to 'a cascade of somatic and psychological experiences that are interpreted through a particular cultural lens'. Western medicine is right to assume that the florid psychological symptoms of Western depression, such as pessimism, self-loathing, and guilt, are generated by the depressive illness itself. But Western medicine fails to acknowledge that without Western culture and the high value it assigns to self-consciousness, there would be no pessimism, self-loathing, and guilt. Depression as defined in DSM-5 is not universal. It is a product of a specifically Western focus on the inner life. Or, as the authors of DSM-5 put it, '[C]linicians should recognize that in most countries the majority of cases of depression go unrecognized in primary care settings and that in many cultures, somatic symptoms are very likely to constitute the presenting complaint.'[13] The authors of the 2008 study argue that in order to understand depression from an intercultural perspective we need to recognize that Western cultures are *cultures* and not some unmarked universal standard from which all other cultures deviate and by which all other cultures must be judged.[14] This is the lesson from cross-cultural psychiatry: we need to recognize that Western depression, and with it the tradition of melancholia, is a culture-bound syndrome. It is a set of mental and physical symptoms that form a recognizable, real disorder, but only within a specific cultural context.

3   National varieties of melancholia in early modern Europe

Some early modern European writers, and needless to say Burton was among them, believed that the whole of Europe was experiencing an epidemic of melancholia.[15] But some writers (often the same ones) claimed that one or other nation either had a special claim to be melancholy or was suffering from its own unique species of melancholia. Could both claims be true? Could melancholia be both a Europe-wide epidemic and a nationally specific one? As long as we think of melancholia as a culture-bound syndrome, this does not pose a problem. On the one hand, by the seventeenth century, melancholia seems to have become nearly universal in Western Europe. Galenic medicine, newly cleansed of medieval scholasticism by the Renaissance humanist scholars and physicians, spread throughout learned Europe, bringing the diagnosis of melancholia with it. Ficino's Neoplatonist theory of melancholy genius took first Italy, then Germany, and then England by storm. The diffusion of ideas was greatly assisted by northern Europeans travelling to Italy, whether to be educated at the Italian universities or to learn from the great Italian artists or simply to take the Grand Tour, which began to be fashionable in the sixteenth century. By the time of Shakespeare's *Hamlet*, Neoplatonism and its doctrine of melancholy genius had become a feature of cultural life at the English court,[16] just as it had earlier at courts right across

---

[13] DSM-5, 166.

[14] Andrew G. Ryder *et al.*, 'The Cultural Shaping of Depression: Somatic Symptoms in China, Psychological Symptoms in North America?', *Journal of Abnormal Psychology* 117 (2008), 300–13 (at p. 310).

[15] Gowland, 'Problem', 77; Midelfort, *History of Madness*, 80, 95.

[16] Babb, *Elizabethan Malady*, 73.

Europe.[17] There was even a mini-epidemic of melancholia in the royal houses of Europe.[18]

On the other hand, regional variants of melancholia were quick to appear. By the seventeenth century it could plausibly be argued that melancholia had increased in incidence in some countries more than others or had taken on particular national forms. This might be attributed to national climatic conditions or socio-political circumstances. Melancholia was perhaps more adaptable to different national environments than any other disease. This was in part because its causes were so various and uncertain, as we saw in the case of melancholia hypochondriaca. If Burton is to be believed, the number of potential causal factors was vast, and this might have added to melancholia's adaptability to national circumstances. It was a simple matter to find a plausible causal factor that was specific to local conditions. In one country the poor climate could be blamed, in another the unhealthy diet, in another social or political factors. Whether these national species of melancholia were real or pretended is, however, another matter altogether. The adaptability of melancholia made it all too easy to construct specious arguments for its national specificity.

The advent of fashionable melancholia in England is usually taken as evidence that the English had a particular susceptibility to the disease, to the extent that melancholia became known as the 'English disease'. (The habit of giving diseases national epithets was a traditional form of cross-border name-calling in early modern Europe: syphilis was variously known as the French disease by most Europeans, the Italian disease by the French, the Spanish disease by the Dutch, and the Polish disease by the Russians.) So powerful was this claim to English ownership of melancholia that George Cheyne could give the title *The English Malady* to his 1733 essay on melancholia, hypochondria, and other 'nervous distempers'. In fact, Cheyne used traditional Galenic arguments. There is little in *The English Malady* that is actually new. But Cheyne was able cleverly to tailor his argument to contemporary English circumstances and to make his English readers feel that something new and unusual was afflicting them – something which *he* understood and could cure. So the traditional attribution of melancholia to the effects of a bad diet, such as we saw in Rufus of Ephesus, becomes for Cheyne a complaint about 'the Richness and Heaviness of our Food'. Cheyne develops this into a broader

---

[17] Marc Fumaroli, 'La Mélancolie et ses remèdes. Classicisme français et maladie de l'âme', in Fumaroli, *La Diplomatie de l'esprit. De Montaigne à La Fontaine* (Paris: Hermann, 1994), 403–39 (at p. 404).

[18] H. C. Erik Midelfort, *Mad Princes of Renaissance Germany* (Charlottesville, VA: University Press of Virginia, 1994).

argument about the pernicious influence of a luxurious lifestyle. England's problem is 'the Wealth and Abundance of the Inhabitants'. Their wealth allows the English to purchase luxury consumables such as coffee, tea, chocolate, and snuff, which are demonstrably bad for the nerves, and for women's nerves in particular.[19] England's wealth and economic success also contributes to the unhealthy living conditions, in particular bad air, which was a notorious cause of diseases going back to Hippocrates' *Airs, Waters, Places*. Cheyne professes to be worried about 'the Humour of Living in great, populous and consequently unhealthy Towns', with London the very worst culprit, the 'greatest, most capacious, close and populous city of the Globe'. Noxious fumes emanate from all the fires, candles, animals, not to mention the mass of people with their 'clouds of stinking breaths and perspiration'.[20] Here the familiar Hippocratic argument about bad air is given a small but significant twist. Whereas Hippocrates was concerned about how different cities were exposed in different ways to the winds, in Cheyne's version the environmental factors responsible for melancholia are man-made, and the danger originates in England's vigorous economic activity. Cheyne also has an argument similar to Rufus' and Ficino's diagnosis of the scholar's melancholia. A significant risk factor is 'the Inactivity and Sedentary Occupations of the better sort [of people]'.[21] In other words, all the causes Cheyne lists belong generically to traditional Hippocratic and Galenic medicine. But Cheyne updates Hippocrates and Galen to take account of the newly discovered physiology of the nerves, and he points the finger at an environment that is the result of English economic progress.

No doubt Cheyne's claims for the specificity of English melancholia were exaggerated, but as a piece of folk wisdom his argument proved remarkably tenacious and long-lived.[22] Soon travellers were finding that its obverse was also true. Where there was no economic progress and no luxury, there could be no melancholia. Travelling in the Highlands of Scotland, Samuel Johnson found the 'natives' blissfully free of melancholia, because, he concluded, they had no leisure time.[23] The compliment that the Scot Cheyne had paid to the English is neatly repaid in the Englishman Johnson's patronizing and presumably ironic compliment to the Scots.

Cheyne's confidently painted picture of an English nation unique in its melancholia soon rigidified into orthodoxy. Melancholia was the English

---

[19] Cheyne, *The English Malady*, 34.   [20] *Ibid.*, 38.   [21] *Ibid.*, i.

[22] Showalter, *Female Malady*, 6–7.

[23] Andrew Solomon, *The Noonday Demon: An Anatomy of Depression* (London: Vintage, 2002), 311.

disease, long before dysfunctional industrial relations and football hooliganism acquired the same label. But this orthodoxy of the English disease simplifies a picture that was in fact more varied. England was by no means alone in laying special claim to melancholia, nor was it the first nation to do so. Spain had a prior claim: the melancholy Spaniard was already proverbial in the sixteenth century.[24] Some said Spain's exceptionally hot, dry climate was to blame.[25] Likewise Venetians were apparently prone to melancholia because they spent too long in the sun.[26] Cheyne would also make this most traditional of causal arguments for English melancholia, though in England's case it was not heat but 'the moisture of our Air' and 'the variableness of our weather' that was to blame. Bishop Berkeley complained of 'the hypochondriac, melancholic complexion' of the Irish, similarly blighted by damp and unpredictable weather.[27] By the early nineteenth century a distinct form of melancholia, or 'chondria', was being claimed by Russians.[28]

Of the European nations, only France, it seems, was considered immune to the climatic causes of melancholia. Louys Pascal de La Court, writing in 1616, claimed that France had an ideal climate and consequently its people enjoyed a perfect constitutional blend of the humours.[29] France, not England, was the exceptional case, and not only on climatic grounds. During the seventeenth-century 'golden age' of melancholia (one of several such golden ages, it should be said), French writers positioned their nation as an exception to the general rule of a European epidemic of melancholia. France was sane and happy. Sometimes a contrast would be drawn between France and its neighbours (and geopolitical enemies) such as Spain, where, according to these French writers, melancholia was rife. This is the argument of La Mothe le Vayer's *Discourse on the Contrariety of the Humours to be Found between Certain Nations, and in Particular between France and Spain* (1636).[30] In 1610 Pierre de Lancre would write off most of Europe as mad, whether because of inconstancy (the Spaniards), heresy (the English), or drunkenness (the Germans).[31] Only France was free of melancholia.

---

[24] Barbara Ehrenreich, *Dancing in the Streets: A History of Collective Joy* (London: Granta, 2007), 131; Klibansky *et al.*, *Saturn and Melancholy*, 234.

[25] Burton, *Anatomy*, vol. I, 234, and Huarte cited by Fumaroli, 'La Mélancolie et ses remèdes', 413.

[26] Hercules de Saxonia cited by Burton, *Anatomy*, vol. I, 234.

[27] George Berkeley, *The Works of George Berkeley, DD, Late Bishop of Cloyne in Ireland : to which is Added an Account of his Life, and Several of his Letters* (Dublin: Exshaw, 1784), 305.

[28] See, for example, Alexander Pushkin, *Eugene Onegin*, trans. Charles Johnson (Harmondsworth: Penguin, 1979), 52.

[29] Fumaroli, 'La Mélancolie et ses remèdes', 415–16.   [30] *Ibid.*, 415–17.

[31] *Ibid.*, 428–9.

In reality the weather had little to do with it and was only a cover for other, usually political agendas. Not least among the advantages of the arguments for national melancholia that we have seen here was to enable a writer to construct an image of his own nation's vigour. In this way melancholia, like so many other ideas, could be mobilized in the formation of early modern national identities. Cheyne was playing a similar game, whether consciously or not. While he appeared to denigrate England for its high incidence of melancholia, he was actually paying his adopted land a backhanded compliment by repeatedly reminding his English readers of their economic achievements. (Cheyne was born in Aberdeen before Scotland's forced union with England.) In any case, just as Cheyne's claims for a uniquely English disease were exaggerated, so too were French claims to be uniquely immune to melancholia. To judge by the frequency of its appearance in French literature in the eighteenth century, melancholia was just as common in France as elsewhere.[32] If we want an explanation for the efforts made by French writers to deny the fact that melancholia was no less endemic in France than in the rest of Europe, we could do worse than look to religion. The French 'war on sadness' was a reaction to France's sixteenth-century religious wars.[33] After its bout of religious madness France would try to rebuild itself as a nation of blooming mental health.

4   Puritan religious melancholia

Did the seventeenth-century French have any legitimate grounds for thinking themselves exceptional? Certainly, there were some very real differences between national melancholias in early modern Europe, as distinct from the specious differences claimed on the basis of climate. As the example of France suggests, the differences resulted in some part from the paths that nations took out of the great age of Christian schism in the sixteenth century. The precise nature of the link between religious schism and melancholia is a vexed issue. But one undisputed fact is that the diffusion of melancholia across Europe occurred during the same period as the great schismatic age of the Reformation and the subsequent religious wars. Understandably, melancholia and religious conflict became connected in the minds of many Europeans.[34]

---

[32] Fritz Schalk, 'Der Artikel "mélancolie" in der Diderot'schen *Enzyklopädie*', in Schalk, *Studien zur französischen Aufklärung* (Frankfurt/Main: Klostermann, 1977), 206–20 (at pp. 213–20).

[33] Fumaroli, 'La Mélancolie et ses remèdes', 412.   [34] Gowland, 'Problem', 118–19.

Among the different regional forms of melancholia, some were certainly connected with the experience of dislocation and trauma suffered during the religious troubles of the sixteenth and seventeenth centuries. A distinctive form of melancholia evolved among the Puritans of New England, who had fled religious persecution in Europe. This and related forms of melancholia were termed 'religious melancholy' by contemporaries, after Burton coined the term in his *Anatomy of Melancholy*. The idea of a link between melancholia and religion had circulated in antiquity and the Middle Ages, though it was not a formally defined species or subspecies of melancholia. Rufus had identified excessive thinking as a cause of melancholia and discussed the case of a melancholic student of geometry.[35] Isḥāq ibn ʿImrān commented on the dangers of excessive longing for God.[36] Indeed, religious melancholia can be understood as a form of love melancholia, a passionate love of God that has been misdirected and corrupted.[37] Until Burton, however, religion was just one of the many potential causes of melancholia and was not differentiated from the others. Burton was the first to make religious melancholia a disease in its own right. In Latinized medical form, the diagnosis of melancholia religiosa was added to the medical taxonomies of the eighteenth century,[38] and it continued to appear in textbooks and encyclopedias well into the nineteenth, until it was gradually replaced by religious mania.[39]

Burton's particular target was Calvinist Puritanism. Adopting Rufus's observation that melancholics can have the gift of prophesy in dreams, Burton criticized the Puritans as false prophets.[40] The charge of religious melancholia against the Puritans was well made in a second sense. Calvinism tended towards a style of morbid and despairing self-scrutiny, of which the writings of Puritan divines and laymen provide ample testimony.[41] Calvin insisted that God had not only predestined true believers for salvation; he had also predestined the reprobate for damnation.[42] This raised the stakes considerably for the uncertain believer. A Calvinist would, of course, want to be absolutely sure of her or his salvation. The activity of 'discerning the spirit' aimed at finding signs of true

---

[35] Rufus, *On Melancholy*, 69.   [36] Isḥāq ibn ʿImrān, *Maqāla fī'l-mālīḫūliyā*, 14.

[37] Gowland, *Worlds*, 70.

[38] Alexander Crichton, *An Inquiry into the Nature and Origin of Mental Derangement*, 2 vols. (London: T. Cadell, W. Davies, 1798), vol. II, 240.

[39] See, for example, Pierer, *Universal-Lexikon*, vol. VII, 86.

[40] Burton, *Anatomy*, vol. III, 386–8.

[41] John Stachniewski, *The Persecutory Imagination: English Puritanism and the Literature of Religious Despair* (Oxford University Press, 1991), 27.

[42] *Ibid.*, 19.

conversion.[43] This search for signs was often conducted in a mood of despair that non-Puritans could easily diagnose as melancholia. The relentless self-scrutiny conducted by Calvinists seemed to conform to an established pattern of melancholic rumination. A successful conversion might even add to this impression by isolating the new convert from the non-Puritan community in a way that also seemed melancholic. (Rufus said that melancholics sought solitude.) Understandably, the Puritans themselves rejected the label of melancholia, which threatened to turn their spiritual struggles into a medical pathology. But their actions belied these denials. The Calvinists played out their melancholia in great psychological detail, documenting their exposure to temptation by imitating the travails of Christ.[44]

The distinctive New England form of religious melancholia added another element: the hardship suffered by the first Pilgrim Fathers in the vast, desolate American landscape, as it appeared to seventeenth-century European eyes.[45] Desolate, pathless wilderness was a traditional element in the iconography of melancholia, as we will see in Chapter 5. The pseudo-Aristotelian *Problems* quotes lines from the *Iliad* describing the solitary wanderings of Bellerophontes across the pathless plain of Aleïon.[46] The tendency of melancholics to seek solitude is noted in most early modern accounts of melancholia. Some authors claimed that desolate places caused melancholia: 'desart places cause melancholy in an instant', says Burton.[47] Not directly related to melancholia, but in some ways analogous to it, early Christian desert hermits had developed the notion of *acedia*, literally a lack of care (Ancient Greek *kēdos*: care, concern) – that is to say, a lethargic neglect of or indifference to the ordained rituals of monastic life. Just as Christ was tempted by Satan in the desert, so the desert hermits could be tempted by the 'noonday demon' of *acedia* and, if they succumbed, would become indifferent to rituals of worship such as prayer.[48] Old Testament texts could also be adduced, such as Psalms 107:4: 'They wandred in the wildernes, in a solitary way: they found no citie to dwell in.' For the New England Puritans this text became palpable. Like their Old Testament forebears, the New England Puritans were fated to wander in places of desolation. The Old Testament texts generated many more texts in

[43] Julius H. Rubin, *Religious Melancholy and Protestant Experience in America* (Oxford University Press, 1994), 30.

[44] John Owen King III, *The Iron of Melancholy: Structures of Spiritual Conversion from the Puritan Conscience to Victorian Neurosis* (Middletown, CT: Wesleyan University Press, 1983), 15.

[45] Rubin, *Religious Melancholy*, 46.   [46] Homer, *Iliad*, 6, 200–3.

[47] Burton, *Anatomy*, vol. I, 237.   [48] Wenzel, *The Sin of Sloth*, 5.

turn.[49] The Puritan spiritual autobiographies that began to appear from the 1630s documented a distinctive American experience of melancholia. Central to this was the theme of migration to the wastelands of America, fraught with danger and uncertainty and filled with the potential of temptation and salvation for the Puritan soul.[50]

5   The disease of nostalgia

Another instance of a regionally distinct form of melancholia is afforded by the early history of nostalgia.[51] First named in a medical dissertation of 1688 by Johannes Hofer, 'Dissertatio medica de nostalgia, oder Heimwehe' (*Medical dissertation on nostalgia, or homesickness*), nostalgia began life as a disease peculiar to Swiss mercenary soldiers. The poverty of Switzerland forced many young men to seek their fortunes abroad. This turned into a semi-organized national industry, with whole companies of Swiss being employed by foreign armies. Swiss companies – 'Switzers', as they were known in English – were proverbial for their ferocity and effective tactics, using the long pike in close formations that were hard to break down. So disciplined and loyal were the troops that they were also employed as guards by foreign courts: the Vatican's Pontifical Swiss Guard became the most famous of these companies. Swiss guards served widely across Europe and even in North America. But removal from their homeland came at a significant cost to the Switzers' mental well-being, and consequently to their employers' purses. In part this was a function of cultural foreignness, and in part it resulted from the difference in landscapes: the contrast of their native mountains to the foreign flatlands where they fought. According to Hofer, the symptoms of nostalgia, or the Swiss disease as it became known, included 'a continuing melancholy, incessant thinking of home, disturbed sleep or insomnia, weakness, loss of appetite, anxiety, cardiac palpitations, stupor, and fever'.[52] There were reports of it ending in death.

Nostalgia was given formal medical recognition not least because of its military significance. Anything that impaired their armies' performance was of grave concern to early modern governments. The most pressing concern was the risk of mass desertion by the financially and militarily valuable Switzers. In his *Dictionary of Music* of 1767, Jean-Jacques

---

[49] King, *Iron of Melancholy*, 13–14.   [50] Rubin, *Religious Melancholy*, 46.

[51] See Simon Bunke, *Heimweh, Studien zur Kultur- und Literaturgeschichte einer tödlichen Krankheit* (Freiburg: Rombach, 2009).

[52] George Rosen, 'Nostalgia: A "Forgotten" Psychological Disorder', *Psychological Medicine* 5 (1975), 340–54 (at p. 341).

Rousseau cites the Swiss herdsmen's songs (*ranz-des-vaches* or *Kuhreihen*) as a prime example of the psychological effects of music. The songs were so beloved of the Switzers and made them so powerfully aware of their distant homeland that their commanders forbade the mercenaries from singing them on pain of death, lest they 'burst into tears, desert or die, so ardent was the desire excited in them to see their country once more'.[53] Like other forms of melancholia, acute nostalgia was activated and exacerbated by an unhappy consciousness of self, in this case a self that was embedded in memories of home. Banning the *Kuhreihen* was a way to block off the consciousness of self that caused the illness to become acute. Rufus, we will recall, had offered a similar prescription. Patients in the early stages of melancholia should not be told their diagnosis, lest this focus their minds on themselves and so lead to more advanced forms of the disease.[54]

In the medical literature of the eighteenth century and in the new specialization of military medicine, nostalgia began to appear with frequency. Two developments are noteworthy. Once nostalgia became widely known, it was given a place in general medical classificatory schemes, and it ceased to be primarily a Swiss or indeed a military problem. Nostalgia became a medical complaint that could affect anyone, like melancholia. Admittedly, different medical authorities classified it in different ways. In view of the nature of its symptoms, there was an obvious logic in classifying it as a subspecies of melancholia, as the German physician Rudolph August Vogel did.[55] Once it was classified within an existing category, nostalgia inevitably lost some of its distinctiveness, since it now shared features with its related diseases. At the same time nostalgia was increasingly being diagnosed in other circumstances than those of the Swiss mercenaries. For instance, Theodor Zwinger defined nostalgia as a general phenomenon, a complaint that 'attacks those who are abroad and cannot accommodate themselves to foreign manners'.[56] In the late eighteenth century there was a spate of cases of homesick female domestic servants, some with awful consequences, such as setting fire to their employers' houses or killing their children. Applied more generally, nostalgia came to be viewed as less acute. Eventually it would acquire a non-medical sense and become a mere mood or feeling, much as

[53] Jean-Jacques Rousseau, *Dictionnaire de Musique*, in *Collection complète des oeuvres de J. J. Rousseau*, ed. Pierre-Alexandre du Peyrou and Paul Moultou (Geneva: Société Typographique, 1780–9), vol. IX, 443 (my translation).
[54] Rufus, *On Melancholy*, 53.   [55] Jackson, *Melancholia*, 377.
[56] Quoted in Joep Leerssen, 'Sublime Landscape and National Character', in Gisela Holfter, Marieke Krajenbrink, and Edward Moxon-Browne (eds.), *Beziehungen und Identitäten: Österreich, Irland und die Schweiz* (Bern: Lang, 2004), 25–35 (at pp. 30–1).

melancholia did when it evolved into non-medical melancholy. From around 1930 nostalgia ceased to be counted as an illness. It was certainly no longer such a pressing concern for the military authorities. Their attention was now focused on other syndromes such as the shell shock of soldiers in the Great War and later the post-traumatic stress disorder of Vietnam veterans.

6   Culture-bound syndromes

In the last two sections, I have tried to make a distinction between plausible and implausible claims that special types of melancholia existed in early modern Europe. The types attributed to local climatic or socio-economic conditions seem to me generally implausible. Depressing though the weather in the British Isles might sometimes be, there seems no good reason to believe that it gave rise to a special form of British or Irish melancholia. Equally, the economic success of eighteenth-century Britain is unlikely to have produced melancholia on an epidemic scale. Conversely, there is no good reason to believe the claims of French writers that France was some-how immune to melancholia. All of these claims for special status seem to me specious. It seems to me that they were most likely motivated, whether directly or indirectly, by the imperatives of nation-building.

On the other hand, it seems to me that there was some substance behind nostalgia and Calvinist religious melancholia, though many individual cases may have been more the product of fashionable imitation than authentic suffering. These latter culturally specific subtypes of melancholia – that is, the *non-specious* subtypes – show how geographical and historical factors can shape the forms taken by mental disorders. Indeed, I want to propose that early modern religious melancholia and Swiss nostalgia can be understood as culture-bound syndromes. In the Introduction, I suggested that Ian Hacking's discussion of fugue offered a good theoretical model for the ways in which cultural factors operate on psychiatric nosology. Hacking's model draws on ideas from biology and engineering. Biological species evolve in ecological spaces called 'niches'. A niche is essentially the sum of the forces determining the reproductive success of an organism: the ecological space in which an organism successfully reproduces. Hacking combines this with the engineering concept of the 'vector'. Vectors are the many and different physical forces that act on a body. Transferred to the biological domain, vectors are the constituent forces that make up the niche.[57] In Hacking's sense, a niche is created by the action of a number of

---

[57] Hacking, *Mad Travellers*, 80–101.

vectors. Hacking uses this model to explain how transient mental disorders can appear and disappear; a mental disorder can be diagnosed for a period of several years, and then it can disappear. A mental disorder can be transient because its niche is a window that is only open temporarily. Individual vectors are constantly changing; in response to these changes the diagnosis must either change itself or cease to exist. This is not to say that in Hacking's transient mental disorders the diseases are *unreal*. Hacking thinks fugue is a plausible way to be mentally ill within a particular cultural niche.[58]

How can Hacking's model be applied to religious melancholia and nostalgia? The niches that allowed these forms of melancholia to flourish were formed from two types of vector: cultural and nosological. The New England Puritans brought a pre-existing diagnosis of melancholia with them from Europe. The peculiar character of American religious melancholia derived from the struggle of the Pilgrim Fathers with their environment, the 'desert' of the American wilderness. This existential struggle was recast in terms drawn from the Old Testament. Cast out from Europe, as it seemed to them, they were, like the Israelites, both chosen by God and sorely tested by Him. This peculiar form of melancholia became less appealing as Americans' attitudes to their land changed from fear to familiarity. At the same time the nosology of melancholia was changing. In place of traditional melancholia with its genial and enthusiastic features, weakness and debility were beginning to be emphasized, and asthenia was on the rise. Asthenia was less amenable to use in a religious context. A diagnosis of 'religious asthenia' would have made little sense, whether in terms of the model of asthenic illness or in terms of religious experience. However, religion did continue to appear in psychiatric classifications, and religion could still be a defining feature of mental illness, but now it would more often be classified as a form of mania.

Nostalgia owed its existence to the move towards formal classificatory systems in the late seventeenth and eighteenth centuries. This created space for various subtypes of melancholia. The initial spark for nostalgia was the experience of Swiss soldiers, and military psychiatry remained an important context for the diagnosis of nostalgia. However, increasingly from the middle of the nineteenth century, and then devastatingly in World War I, the nature of war changed. The terrors of mass, mechanized warfare imposed new and more acute stresses on the minds of soldiers, and the attention of military psychiatrists shifted to battlefield shock. Thus, while the social conditions for a diagnosis of nostalgia remained,

---

[58] Hacking's view is actually rather more complex than my bald summary suggests: see Hacking, *Mad Travellers*, 80–102.

as people continued to move from their homelands in search of work, nostalgia ceased to be a formal medical diagnosis.

Aside from these subtypes, the argument of this book is that melancholia more generally can be understood as a culture-bound syndrome. Historically, melancholia has been an experience of people in the West more or less consistently since antiquity. In terms of nosology, the existence of melancholia depends on the categories and methods established by Graeco-Roman medicine. As for cultural vectors, comparison with non-Western forms of mental illness suggests that melancholia is dependent on a peculiar feature of Western culture – namely, the exceptionally high value that Western culture assigns to inwardness and self-consciousness. In order to demonstrate this satisfactorily, we need a Hacking-style argument about the cultural niche in which melancholia flourished. So we now need to consider how well our model of a melancholia caused by cultures of self-consciousness tallies with the evidence of European cultural history. Can a rise in the value assigned to self-consciousness be linked to the emergence of melancholia? When did this happen? What socio-cultural forces were necessary for melancholia to arise and to persist?

7   Melancholia, depression, and modern capitalism

According to one tradition in Western thought, modernity is a melancholy place. As moderns, we witness the massive forces that forged 'the tremendous cosmos of the modern economic order' (in the words of Max Weber). These are the forces of economic, bureaucratic, political, social, and scientific rationalization. Modernity promised us unrivalled mastery over our world by making it calculable and predictable, but instead of being masters we find ourselves prisoners in the 'iron cage' of economic rationality (Weber again).[59] Weber's prescient view of the melancholy condition of modern man, in the closing pages of his classic *The Protestant Ethic and the Spirit of Capitalism* (1904–5), is supported by some recent research into the social causes of depression. Increasing affluence in the West has made us less happy, not more. Why? Could it be that the recent explosion in diagnoses of depression has been fuelled by the spread of 'turbo-capitalism' and the consequent growth of income inequality in rich nations since the 1980s?[60] Studies of income inequality do seem to

---

[59] Max Weber, *The Protestant Ethic and the Spirit of Capitalism*, trans. Talcott Parsons, with an introduction by Anthony Giddens (London: Routledge, 1992), 123.
[60] The term 'turbo-capitalism' was coined by Edward Luttwak, *Turbo-Capitalism: Winners and Losers in the Global Economy* (New York: HarperCollins, 1999).

confirm this claim. Income inequality appears to have an adverse effect on mental health. This may be because high levels of income inequality make people more anxious about their own status in society (status anxiety). Alternatively, income inequality may reduce social cohesion. As income inequality rises, social cohesion diminishes as people lose trust in others and in social institutions.[61]

While there is some evidence that the growing gap between rich and poor makes people depressed, other data make the picture more complex. Status anxiety is a function of relative poverty, but a number of studies have shown that *absolute* poverty on its own is a major causal factor in depression.[62] US welfare recipients are three times more likely to suffer from depression than those not on welfare.[63] A link between poverty and depression makes perfect sense, but it is less clear what the nature of the link is. Does poverty cause depression or does depression cause poverty? (This question of causal relations will also turn out to be especially thorny in the case of melancholia.) One can imagine that depression among the poor might be self-selecting. People with depression might drift into positions of social exclusion, because, for instance, their depression makes them unable to find or stay in employment. But studies following the course of depression over time have found that unemployment is more likely to precede the onset of depression than follow it. This suggests that in the majority of cases people become depressed as a result of poverty, before becoming even poorer as a result of their depression.[64] Conversely, it may be that affluence actually confers some protection against depression, perhaps because affluence brings higher self-esteem, in which case the social anxiety thesis would be hard to sustain. In the UK, people in local authority housing are more likely to suffer from poor mental health

---

[61] Richard Layte, 'The Association Between Income Inequality and Mental Health: Testing Status Anxiety, Social Capital, and Neo-Materialist Explanations', *European Sociological Review* 28 (2011), 498–511.

[62] For a general discussion of poverty and depression, see John W. Lynch, George A. Kaplan, and Sarah J. Shema, 'Cumulative Impact of Sustained Economic Hardship on Physical, Cognitive, Psychological, and Social Functioning', *New England Journal of Medicine* 337 (1997), 1889–95.

[63] Krista K. Olson and LaDonna Pavetti, 'Personal and Family Challenges to the Successful Transition from Welfare to Work' (www.urban.org/publications/406850.html).

[64] S. M. Montgomery *et al.*, 'Unemployment Predates Symptoms of Depression and Anxiety Resulting in Medical Consultation in Young Men', *International Journal of Epidemiology* 28 (1999), 95–100; D. Dooley, R. Catalano, and G. Wilson, 'Depression and Unemployment: Panel Findings from the Epidemiologic Catchment Area study', *American Journal of Community Psychology* 22 (1994), 745–65; S. H. Wilson and G. M. Walker, 'Unemployment and Health: A Review', *Public Health* 107 (1993), 153–62.

than those who own their property.[65] It may be that people suffering from poverty are exposed to more mental and physical stress. Damp, run-down, insecure, or noisy accommodation has also been linked to higher levels of depression.[66] Perhaps the impact of poverty on depression is indirect and works through some mediating factor. Poor living conditions can cause poor physical health, which in turn can lead to depression.[67] Other factors such as the lack of social support networks, poor educational attainment, and a tedious, unpleasant, or poorly paid job may also play a role.[68]

Research into the economic causes of depression seems to show that both extreme affluence and poverty (but also in some circumstances being somewhere in between) can be depressogenic. This makes it hard to believe that the material conditions of people's lives directly determine their susceptibility to depression: how could good and bad living conditions both have the same effect? There are two ways out of this bind. It is possible that depression might be a multicausal disorder. Perhaps there are many types of depressogenic stress that are triggered by different, even antithetical situations. Or maybe levels of wealth and educational attainment determine not *whether* people become depressed but the *ways* in which they become depressed. Some evidence suggests that the poor and the rich experience depression differently. A US study by Opler and Small found that poor people tended to experience emotional symptoms. Poor women reported these in bodily terms, while poor men tended to complain of their inability to cope with life situations. Wealthy patients, on the other hand, were more likely to express disenchantment with social aspects of their lives. Differences also made themselves felt in how people were treated. Poor people who received treatment were more likely to be prescribed medication, whereas wealthy patients considered medication inferior to psychotherapeutic treatments. (The study was conducted in

---

[65] G. Lewis et al., 'Socioeconomic Status, Standard of Living, and Neurotic Disorder', *Lancet* 352 (1998), 605–9; H. Meltzer et al., *The Prevalence of Psychiatric Morbidity Among Adults Living in Private Households* (London: OPCS, 1995).

[66] J. L. Hopton and S. M. Hunt, 'Housing Conditions and Mental Health in a Disadvantaged Area in Scotland', *Journal of Epidemiology and Community Health* 50 (1996), 56–61.

[67] Meltzer et al., *Prevalence*; R. Gomm, 'Mental Health and Inequality', in *Mental Health Matters – A Reader*, ed. T. Heller et al. (Basingstoke: Open University Press, 1996), 110–20.

[68] See, for instance, Gomm, 'Mental Health'; D. Baker and H. Taylor, 'The Relation Between Condition-Specific Morbidity, Social Support and Material Deprivation in Pregnancy and Early Motherhood', *Social Science and Medicine* 45 (1997), 1325–36; R. A. Schoevers et al., 'Risk Factors for Depression in Later Life: Results of a Prospective Community Based Study', *Journal of Affective Disorders* 59 (2000), 127–37; Meltzer et al., *Prevalence*.

1968 and so predated the middle-class fashion for SSRIs by some years.)[69]

What most of these studies omit to discuss is the mentality and cultural environment of their subjects. As the 2008 study of Chinese and US depression suggests, mentalities are crucial to the way mental disorders are formed, both in the way they are experienced by sufferers and the way medical science formulates disorder constructs. So while the statistics on income inequality might appear compelling, the case itself remains largely speculative.

Weber's classic essay is much more subtle and carefully argued, though it is with subsequent (and arguably simplified) versions of his argument that we will be concerned here. Weber was interested in constructing a sociological typology of early modern mentalities. Subsequently, his ideas were taken up by historians who were more concerned to see how socio-economic changes in early modern Europe led to changes in mentalities, among which was the epidemic of melancholia. This latter question is what interests us here, not so much the social-typological one asked by Weber. Another inspiration for historians has been Jacob Burckhardt's *The Civilization of the Renaissance in Italy* (1860). Burckhardt argued that a new form of individualism marked the threshold between the Middle Ages and the early modern period. In the second part of Burckhardt's book, 'The Development of the Individual', he claimed to find a clean break between medieval and modern concepts of the self. Modernity begins with a shift from a corporate identity to a personal identity:

In the Middle Ages . . . man was conscious of himself only as a member of a race, people, party, family, or corporation – only through some general category. In [Renaissance] Italy . . . man became a spiritual *individual*, recognized himself as such. . . At the close of the thirteenth century Italy began to swarm with individuality; the ban laid upon human personality was dissolved; and a thousand figures meet us each in its own special shape and dress. . . The Italians of the fourteenth century knew little of false modesty or of hypocrisy in any shape; not one of them was afraid of singularity, or being and seeming unlike his neighbours.[70]

Burckhardt seems to be unaware of melancholia and barely mentions Ficino.[71] His portrayal of Renaissance individualism contains no pathological elements, unlike Weber's 'iron cage'. Nonetheless, Burckhardt's theory of the emergence of individualism lies behind many attempts to

[69] Marvin K. Opler and S. Mouchly Small, 'Cultural Variables Affecting Somatic Complaints and Depression', *Psychosomatics: Journal of Consultation and Liaison Psychiatry* 9 (1968), 261–6.

[70] Jacob Burckhardt, *The Civilization of the Renaissance in Italy* (Harmondsworth: Penguin, 1990), 98–9.

[71] *Ibid.*, 146, 328.

account for early modern melancholia. (Some of these will be discussed in the following sections.) Moreover, as I hope to show in the following pages, Burckhardt's theory is the source of one of their major flaws. The next sections deal with questions of historical causation. Why did the supposed early modern epidemic of melancholia happen? Or in Ian Hacking's terms, what were the features of early modern culture that made melancholia an acceptable way to be mad? Would something like Burckhardt's individualism or Weber's 'iron cage' be plausible candidates for the vectors forming the niche occupied by melancholia?

8   The 'Weber–Tawney' thesis and early modern melancholia

Weber's starting point was the observation that in early modern Europe capital appeared to be disproportionately in the hands of Protestants. (This is now generally considered to be untrue.)[72] This came about, Weber argued, because the capitalist and Protestant belief systems were broadly congruent and shared some important features. Early modern capitalism's guiding idea was the accumulation of money, not for any purpose, but for its own sake and without any thought to enjoy its fruits.[73] There was an ascetic element in early capitalism. Making money was a calling, an ethical imperative, an end in itself. Weber believed that this notion of a calling, a divine sanction for the pursuit of a worldly goal, was also central to Protestantism. Luther asked that we accept our life in this world as a task.[74] The worldly asceticism of the Protestant calling was further heightened by Calvin's doctrine of predestination. Calvin himself was happily convinced of his own salvation, but for his followers things were not so easy. Predestination caused intense feelings of loneliness. Your salvation was a matter for you, and nobody else had any part in it.[75] The sensuous elements of religion and culture were empty blandishments. Equally, self-scrutiny was regarded by many Calvinists as self-indulgent, though many still felt the need to engage in painfully microscopic self-scrutiny. You might scrutinize your soul for signs of conversion, but the only way to be sure was to work at your worldly calling, by prospering as a capitalist, for instance. In this way you could create in yourself the confidence that you would be saved.[76]

In his account of capitalism and Calvinism, Weber presented a picture of two broadly congruent belief systems. Historians writing after Weber have had concerns about the model of historical causation they claimed to

---

[72] Weber, *Protestant Ethic*, xxii.   [73] *Ibid.*, 53.   [74] *Ibid.*, 47.   [75] *Ibid.*, 60.   [76] *Ibid.*, 69.

find in his work. In his preface to the 1930 translation of Weber's essay, the economic historian R. H. Tawney criticized what he perceived as Weber's suggestion that Protestantism caused capitalism.[77] From an economic historian's point of view, this seemed to put the cart before the horse. In some parts of Europe capitalism had already developed prior to the Reformation, and Weber seemed to have overlooked this. In his 1926 *Religion and the Rise of Capitalism*, Tawney expanded on his critique of Weber, albeit in a manner broadly sympathetic to Weber's aims. Tawney agreed that capitalism and Protestantism were congruent systems, but he argued that capitalism was chiefly created by large-scale economic movements, and these in turn helped to shape the spirit of Protestantism.[78] The causal flow ran primarily from economic changes to spiritual ones; the development and spread of early modern individualism stemmed from economic not religious roots. Indeed, in some ways, capitalism and religion were in conflict. As capitalism developed, there was increasing resistance to attempts to enforce church morality on economic activity.[79] Religious morality was slowly sidelined, and large areas of economic and social life were now free of religious oversight and stripped of spiritual significance.[80] This loss of religious control over economic life seemed to contribute to people's feelings of unease. For Tawney, therefore, it was the evolution of capitalism, and especially the instability and unrest caused by the move from an agrarian to a mercantile society, that lay behind modern individualism and its distinctive sense of insecurity.[81]

Since Tawney, several variants of the so-called Weber–Tawney thesis have been applied to the problem of early modern melancholia. According to these models, the underlying cause of the epidemic of melancholia was the economic and social uncertainty to which early capitalism led.[82] Within this experience of uncertainty, other smaller-scale causal factors have also been identified: the shortage of routes to advancement for young men in Elizabethan and Jacobean society,[83] the breakdown of the Elizabethan and Jacobean system of literary patronage under economic pressures,[84] and the end of mass expressions of happiness and the

[77] R. H. Tawney, 'Preface' in Max Weber, *The Protestant Ethic and the Spirit of Capitalism*, trans. Talcott Parsons (London: Allen & Unwin, 1930), 7–8.
[78] R. H. Tawney, *Religion and the Rise of Capitalism: A Historical Study* (London: Murray, 1926), 319–21.
[79] *Ibid.*, 186.   [80] *Ibid.*, 188.   [81] *Ibid.*, 137.
[82] Erich Fromm, *Fear of Freedom* (London: Routledge, 2001).
[83] L. C. Knights, 'Seventeenth-Century Melancholy', *Criterion* 13 (1933–4), 97–112.
[84] Vieda Skultans, *English Madness: Ideas on Insanity, 1580–1890* (London: Routledge & Kegan Paul, 1979), 21.

increasing regulation of the individual that resulted from capitalist rationalization.[85]

As plausible as each of these arguments is, there are two weaknesses in the underlying Weber–Tawney thesis, at least insofar as early modern melancholia is concerned. One is social, the other conceptual. The social problem takes us back to the causal question that we discussed earlier in this section: how do socio-economic factors cause mental disorders? To judge by the arguments of Weber's successors, melancholia was a disease of the upper and aspiring middle classes: Calvinist aristocratic grandees and wealthy burghers, landowners, the commercial classes, and the nobles and hangers-on at court. These groups would be the most sensitive barometers of the unsettling experiences of emergent capitalism and of the first stirrings of individualism. And they would be the first to experience melancholia.

While there is evidence that melancholia was more common in the upper levels of society, the reasons for this had little to do with economics and much more to do with the status of melancholia as a fashionable disease. The fashionable standing of melancholia seems to have been established first in the Italian cities, above all Florence, where Ficino rediscovered the pseudo-Aristotelian *Problems* XXX/1 and formulated the doctrine of Neoplatonic melancholy genius. Once melancholia was established as a status marker, the Italian elite jealously guarded it from people of lower status.[86] The association of melancholia with high status may also be at the root of the strange mini-epidemic of melancholia among the princes of the Holy Roman Empire.[87] A Tuscan legate visiting the court of Rudolf II in Vienna in 1609 commented that Rudolf seemed 'disturbed in his mind by some ailment of melancholy, he has begun to love solitude and shut himself off in his palace as if behind the bars of a prison'.[88] In instances of this kind there is no sign of the impact of Calvinism or capitalism. More likely culprits are the courtly culture of Renaissance humanism, with its Neoplatonic and occult obsessions.

The patchy distribution of melancholia across society confirms the role that fashion played in its diffusion. The case notebooks of Richard Napier, himself an occultist,[89] support the conclusion that melancholia was more common in the higher social strata, but again this was due to its being a fashionable disease.[90] In John Lyly's comedy *Midas* (1592), a page

---

[85] Ehrenreich, *Dancing in the Streets*.   [86] Klibansky *et al.*, *Saturn*, 251.

[87] Midelfort, *Mad Princes*.

[88] R. J. W. Evans, *Rudolf II and His World: A Study in Intellectual History, 1576–1612* (Oxford University Press, 1973), 45.

[89] Macdonald, *Mystical Bedlam*, 16.   [90] *Ibid.*, 34–5.

describes melancholia as 'the creast of courtiers armes'.[91] Like other fashions, melancholia came to be a way of distinguishing yourself from less elite social groups. Often the diagnosis of melancholia among Napier's gentlefolk was prompted by the patients themselves, who came to Napier with a preformed self-diagnosis of melancholia, precisely because they knew it was a socially desirable label. Members of the lower classes, on the other hand, were criticized for pretending to be melancholics. For these patients Napier tended to prefer the diagnosis of 'troubled in mind' or 'mopish'.[92]

The diffusion of fashionable melancholia was also aided by the international character of elite culture in the early modern period. Ficino's writings on melancholia, written in Latin, of course, were accessible to all learned Europeans. Another means of diffusion was the grand tour, which helped to bring Neoplatonic melancholia to London. Melancholia could also travel with luxury goods, whose wealthy users in eighteenth-century England were more likely to be 'People of Condition'.[93] Witness Cheyne's theory of the luxury-induced 'English Malady'.

Initially, therefore, melancholia seems to have been a disease of the affluent, and its spread was occasioned more by its fashionable status than by capitalist individualism. Although its origins were in elite culture, melancholia did spread beyond the European elites. Here again capitalist individualism is by no means the most obvious explanation. Having claimed melancholia as 'the creast of courtiers armes', Lyly's page laments that 'now every base companion ... sayes he is melancholy'.[94] Fashions flow down through society more quickly than wealth. And no exceptional wealth is needed for a person to behave like a melancholic. Melancholia was also diagnosed in places and social groups well beyond the reach of courtly fashion. There is evidence of melancholia among the lower classes in relatively backward rural communities – in other words, among people who were initially least affected by the growth of capital or the rise of individualism or urban fashions. The Puritan divine Richard Baxter (1615–1691) complained that he was called on to give spiritual physic to 'a multitude of melancholly Persons from several Parts of the Land, some of high Quality, some of low, some very exquisitely learned, some unlearned'.[95] In the villages around Reformation Zurich, melancholia was reported among Calvinist craftsmen and manual workers. In adopting the Reformed religion, they would abandon their communities' traditional religious beliefs and engage instead in the demanding routines of

[91] Quoted in Babb, *Elizabethan Malady*, 78.   [92] Macdonald, *Mystical Bedlam*, 151–3.
[93] Sena, *Melancholic Madness*, 294.   [94] Quoted in Babb, *Elizabethan Malady*, 78.
[95] Quoted in Gowland, 'Problem', 78.

dialogue with a personal God and living an exemplary Christian life. In the process they might be excluded from the village community, their consequent isolation being a potential cause of melancholia. These cases do little to support a Tawney-style link between Calvinism and capitalist acquisitiveness. If there was a link between hard work and melancholia, it was more that Calvinist ministers wisely advised their mentally distressed flock to commit themselves to activity as a cure for their melancholia.[96]

If some physicians like Napier were disinclined to diagnose ordinary folk as melancholics, other physicians had no such qualms and treated the poor according to the best Galenic practice. The sad or idle poor did sometimes receive appropriate and sympathetic medical help. The melancholy poor were not locked up on grounds of fecklessness. The picture of a mass internment of the poor painted by Michel Foucault is not borne out by the evidence.[97] Of course, ordinary folk would rarely gain access to learned physicians, and the traditional forms of healing for mental distress would in most cases be tried first: spiritual physic, blessing, exorcism, traditional herbal preparations, other forms of folk or quack remedies.[98] However, an understanding of the humoral basis of melancholia was not confined to learned physicians and their patients or to the readers of Ficino's Neoplatonic philosophy. Alongside these elite theories of melancholia, there were also folk versions of humoral theory available in chapbooks and all manner of popular medical wisdom.[99] For instance, cases of what appeared to be hereditary melancholia could be explained in terms of 'bad blood' or inherited sin. The eighteenth-century Schmid family from Kloten in the canton of Zurich feared, as a result of several suicides, that melancholia was in their blood or that one of their ancestors must have committed some terrible sin.[100]

. The social picture is complex, and fashionable melancholia alone cannot explain it. Needless to say, the type of melancholia that afflicted the Schmids of Kloten was different from the modish disease of Napier's wealthy patients. Nor was the spread of religious melancholia fanned by the winds of fashion, except insofar as Calvinist self-scrutiny was transmitted by personal contagion and the reading of Calvinist literature. Perhaps there has been too much focus on fashionable melancholia. Ficino's genial melancholia may have achieved a cultural prominence, above all in the works of the poets, far beyond its real incidence among the

---

[96] Markus Schär, *Seelennöte der Untertanen. Selbstmord, Melancholie und Religion im Alten Zürich, 1500–1800* (Zürich: Chronos, 1985), 287–9.

[97] Edward Shorter, *A History of Psychiatry: From the Era of the Asylum to the Age of Prozac* (New York: Wiley, 1997), 5, 16–17.

[98] Kutzer, *Anatomie des Wahnsinns*, 33.   [99] Arikha, *Passions and Tempers*, 86–7.

[100] Schär, *Seelennöte*, 12.

population, even among the moneyed classes. At the high point of Elizabethan and Jacobean courtly Neoplatonism, elite melancholia was more commonly seen as a dangerous and damaging disease than a fashion statement. Melancholia attracted opprobrium and stigma.[101] Many were critical of the Neoplatonic view of melancholia, initially on moral grounds, though in the later seventeenth century genial melancholia was also dismissed as irrational.[102] In sixteenth-century Germany, for instance, as magic and witchcraft were gradually displaced by an obsession with demonology, melancholia too came to be 'demonized' by the intelligentsia.[103] As it was stigmatized, melancholia became serviceable as a form of slander. The elite might see melancholia as socially suspect. Puritans were widely stigmatized as religious melancholics, and through these accusations elites were often merely expressing their fear of lower-class disorder.[104] (The accusation of melancholia was part of a wider tradition of psychologizing non-conformist beliefs which dated back to the early Reformation. The Anabaptists were singled out for special treatment and widely derided as insane and melancholic.)[105] Even if the non-conformists were, in fact, not plebeian rabble, it could still be effective to characterize them as such. But escape from the stigma of lower-class melancholia was also possible. There are striking cases of religious melancholics who ascended from poverty to relative comfort, and for whom melancholia's association with artistic creativity and prophetic inspiration – precisely the elements of melancholia that were traditionally the preserve of the affluent classes – made it an asset on their route to social success.[106] The eighteenth century affords some celebrated cases of poor melancholics who rose to cultural prominence, most notably the 'ploughman poet' Robert Burns and the German novelist, journalist, and erstwhile hatter's apprentice Karl Philipp Moritz, whose literary career was substantially based on melancholia.

Thus, melancholia was distributed widely if patchily through society and was not only the prerogative of social elites, nor was it the property of a particular religious sect or sects. We should be wary of identifying early modern melancholia too closely with Calvinism or Protestantism. We have already seen how non-Calvinists criticized the Calvinists' excessive scrupulosity as religious melancholia. But Catholics also succumbed to

---

[101] The criticisms are documented in Winfried Schleiner, *Melancholy, Genius and Utopia in the Renaissance* (Wiesbaden: Harrassowitz, 1991), *passim*, but especially 31–108.

[102] Schleiner, *Melancholy*, 38–9.   [103] Midelfort, *History of Madness*, 53–4.

[104] Michael Heyd, 'The Reaction to Enthusiasm', *Journal of Modern History* 53 (1981), 258–80 (at pp. 278–9).

[105] See MacCulloch, *The Reformation*, on Luther's abuse of the Zwickau prophets (142) and Calvin's of the Anabaptists (196). See also Gowland, *Worlds*, 159.

[106] Klibansky *et al.*, *Saturn*, 95.

melancholy scrupulosity, especially once the Catholic Church had begun seriously to respond to the Reformation. Major Catholic figures such as Ignatius Loyola (1491–1556), Teresa of Avila (1515–1582), and John of the Cross (1542–1591) diagnosed a dangerous potential for melancholia among Catholic believers. (It was no accident that these were Spaniards. The Spanish melancholia that we noted in section 3 of this chapter was thought by some to be connected with the peculiarly gloomy Spanish strain of Catholicism.) Nor was melancholia only a Christian phenomenon. The medical tradition was pagan in origin. The period produced a wealth of secular, confessional melancholy literature, art, and music.

9   Self-consciousness and individualism

Patchy though it is, evidence for the broad diffusion of melancholia through social groups and religious sects is compelling. This causes a problem for historians in the tradition of Burckhardt, Weber, and Tawney. Its diversity and wide diffusion make early modern melancholia difficult to explain in terms of individualism or capitalism, because for most of the period in question the effects of economic change were quite limited in their social and geographical reach. One might also observe that the versions of the Weber–Tawney thesis advanced by historians of early modern melancholia put too much emphasis on socio-economic factors and too little on the sort of ideal typology elaborated by Weber himself. The diffusion of early modern melancholia was in the first place a diffusion not of economic or social conditions, but of practices of self-scrutiny, chiefly through the medium of religion, philosophy, or literature. These might include various forms of melancholic self-absorption: Calvinist or Catholic scrupulosity; Neoplatonic, astrological, and occult imaginings of selfhood; and literary and other discursive practices focused on the self, such as Renaissance self-fashioning.

What motivated and sustained all of these practices was the belief that self-consciousness was a virtue. The belief was remarkably widespread. It was held by different social and cultural groups for different reasons. The point of access to melancholia and the consequences in terms of personal suffering were not always the same. Nor is it necessary to imagine that all members of a given society signed up to self-consciousness to the same degree; only that significant and prominent parts did so. Nonetheless, belief in the virtue of self-consciousness was a necessary prerequisite of early modern melancholia. In Hacking's terms, the high value accorded to self-consciousness in many circles was one of the primary vectors in the niche in which melancholia flourished. Or if we think of early modern melancholia as a Western culture-bound syndrome, then one specifically

Western cultural artefact that gave rise to early modern melancholia was self-consciousness.[107]

At this point a distinction needs to be made between self-consciousness and individualism. To stress the importance of self-consciousness is to appeal to a narrative of Western history that is both subtly and substantially different from the accounts of the rise of individualism in the West offered by intellectual and cultural historians (e.g. Burckhardt, Charles Taylor, Colin Morris) and historically minded sociologists and anthropologists (e.g. Marcel Mauss). In two respects the histories of self-consciousness and individualism share common ground. Both histories are distinctively and uniquely histories of the West; Western individualism is an exception, an anomaly.[108] Second, a precise distinction between individualism and self-consciousness is no doubt desirable, as, for instance, in the history of philosophy. Consciousness and consciousness of self raise a different set of philosophical problems from individuation and identity, and in the history of philosophy the two sets of problems can be distinguished from one another. For instance, there is a long tradition of reflection on questions of identity – for instance, in medieval philosophy – whereas there is relatively little discussion of consciousness (if we confine ourselves to the word itself and its cognates) until about 1720.[109] However, the broader historical phenomena often represent a blend of individualism and self-consciousness, such that some historians, such as Taylor and Morris, see no need to distinguish between the two. Other historians do make a distinction, and I hope to show in this section why it can be helpful to do so.

We can begin by distinguishing between two aspects of the self. Individualism requires us to think of ourselves as different from other selves. But self in this sense need not imply a focus on interiority. Burckhardt's fourteenth-century Italian individuals were, at least as Burckhardt describes them, not especially interested in their own interiority. For the most part what differentiated these individuals from others was an exterior individuality: talents and possessions and behaviours that were externally manifest. The other sense of self – self as the object of internally focused attention – might also involve individuation; my interiority might be different from

---

[107] On self-consciousness as a Western cultural artefact, see Yi-fu Tuan, *Segmented Worlds and Self: Group Life and Individual Consciousness* (Minneapolis, MN: University of Minnesota Press, 1982), 139.

[108] Charles Taylor, *Sources of the Self: The Making of Modern Identity* (Cambridge, MA: Harvard University Press, 1989), 111; Colin Morris, *The Discovery of the Individual, 1050–1200* (New York: Harper and Row, 1972), 2.

[109] See the excellent discussion in Udo Thiel, *The Early Modern Subject: Self-Consciousness and Personal Identity from Descartes to Hume* (Oxford University Press, 2011), 5–26 and *passim*.

yours. On the other hand, it might be that we share the same kind of interiority, in some respects at least. For instance, the language in which we describe our interiority might share a common vocabulary. In concrete historical terms, I give some examples of this 'communal interiority' below. Some forms of self-consciousness might even be anti-individualistic. Two such cases – religious traditions that were radically self-conscious and at the same time anti-individualistic – are Puritanism and its offshoot German Pietism, both of which, not by accident, are central to the history of melancholia. The Puritans of England and New England developed a strong culture of self-scrutiny, and the German Pietists followed them in this. Puritans examined their souls for signs of conversion, by which they might know whether they were elect or reprobate. In concrete terms this expressed itself in distinctive literary practices – notably, the composition of spiritual autobiographies and devotional literature in very large quantities. So far this seems compatible with the individualism theory of Burckhardt, Weber, and others. But a closer look at the culture of Puritanism shows that individualism was often absent. The routines and practices of Calvinism were communal in nature. Much of the Calvinist and Pietist literature was highly formulaic. It deployed a set of narrative structures and a vocabulary that were distinctively Calvinist-Pietist, but were common property within the sects. Certainly, much of the Calvinist and Pietist literature *appears* individualistic. The appearance can be deceptive. Calvinist and Pietist writings are generally not distinctive at the level of the individual believer so much as at the level of the *community* of believers. When Calvinists and Pietists differentiate themselves from other believers, in the first place they are differentiating themselves from the members of other sects, not from other members of their own sect. So when the German Pietists of the eighteenth century began to produce their own spiritual autobiographies and devotional writings, they took most of their vocabulary from the writings of their Puritan spiritual allies. In fact, some of the ostensibly authentic German Pietist spiritual autobiographies were recycled from English Puritan originals. For instance, Johann Heinrich Reitz's *History of the Reborn* (*Historie der Wiedergebohrenen*), first published in 1698 and one of the most influential collections of pietist autobiographies, was in large part translated from the Welsh Puritan Vavasor Powell's *Spiritual Experiences of Sundry Believers* (1653).[110] Far from being individualistic, Puritans and pietists expressed their self-consciousness in communally created and repeatedly reused forms. In a sense this was of no consequence because, hard as it might be for us to comprehend from our post-Romantic

---

[110] Peter Damrau, *The Reception of English Puritan Literature in Germany* (London: Maney, 2006), 31–4.

perspective, the function of the Puritan and Pietist spiritual autobiography was decidedly *not* to assert the individuality of the writer. On the contrary, the aim was to become part of a community, the community of the elect brethren. The composition and delivery of a spiritual autobiography could even serve as a passport to acceptance into a Puritan congregation. By the 1640s in New England, a requirement for full membership of some Puritan congregations was a written account of the believer's conversion.[111] In this context individualism would have been entirely out of place. The course of a Puritan spiritual autobiography was more likely to involve the elimination of troublesome individualism than its cultivation. This made sense within the socio-political context of Calvinism because Calvinist communities were profoundly anti-individualistic in nature.[112] Weber himself described Calvinism as an 'absolutely unbearable form of ecclesiastical control of the individual'.[113] It can be argued that as a result of the intrusion of religious authorities into the lives of believers, the Reformation led to more conformity and more regulation of the private sphere, not less.[114] Puritans who delivered their spiritual autobiographies to their fellow congregationalists were granting the congregation insight into and control over their spiritual experience.

The examples of Calvinism and Pietism show not only that individualism and self-consciousness are not necessarily the same, but also that they can in some circumstances be opposed to or in conflict with one another. The ambivalent relationship between individualism and self-consciousness was discussed by Lawrence Stone in his study of marriage and sexual practices in early modern England. (Stone's large-scale argument, which has been rightly criticized, is of no concern here; what concerns us is one minor detail of his account.) Stone claimed to discern the rise of an 'affective individualism' in the early modern period. The family developed into what we recognize as the nuclear family, united by bonds of marriage and immediate consanguinity. Early modern Britons began to show a strong sense of individual autonomy. Feelings of sexual guilt began to ebb. The traditions of sharing family space in the home, with grown-up children often sharing their parents' and one another's beds, gave way to a growing demand for physical privacy.[115] For our purposes the key point in Stone's argument is that within this emergent individualism were two tendencies, and that these tendencies were quite distinct. One was a concern with personality; early modern Britons

---

[111] King, *The Iron of Melancholy*, 42.   [112] MacCulloch, *Reformation*, 606.
[113] Weber, *Protestant Ethic*, 37.   [114] MacCulloch, *Reformation*, 634–5.
[115] Lawrence Stone, *The Family, Sex and Marriage in England, 1500–1800*, abridged edition (London: Penguin, 1990), 22.

became concerned with their inwardly original and distinct character as persons. In this sense, individualism betokened an interest in the interiority of selves and a high estimation of self-consciousness. The other tendency was a striving for social autonomy. Like Burckhardt's Renaissance Italians, Stone's early modern Britons demanded that they be allowed to be different, that this difference should be respected, and that society must not intrude too far into their privacy as autonomous individuals. Now, not only were these two tendencies distinct, Stone argues; they also sprang from 'antithetical psychological impulses'.[116] The former type of individualism, in the sense of self-consciousness, stemmed from a need to scrutinize the self for the signs of sin or salvation. One purpose of self-scrutiny, then, was to detect and root out sinfulness; it was a means to discipline the self. The literature of Puritanism is a prime example of this, powered as it was by a 'persecutory imagination'.[117] This form of individualism did not necessarily lead to respect for individual autonomy. In fact, in Calvinist communities, it often led to the opposite, to a 'suspicious and inquisitorial society, constantly on the watch to spy out the sins of others and to suppress all deviations from the true way'.[118]

To say that Puritanism was instinctively anti-individualistic is not to deny it any individualism at all. Puritan communities were, of course, famously schismatic and prone to split into ever smaller communities of 'true believers'. (Religious communities in contemporary North America continue to provide evidence of this.) These continual schisms might be interpreted as evidence of an individualistic tendency. Yet they might with equal justice be interpreted as evidence of the intolerable lack of opportunities for individual expression within religious communities, which creates such powerful tensions between members that some feel they have no choice but to splinter off.

Just as self-consciousness could exist without individualism, so too individualism was possible without self-consciousness. One such instance is the individualism that Burckhardt found in the Italian Renaissance. This was more a socio-political than a cultural phenomenon, even if it did have profound cultural consequences.[119] Burckhardt argued that the efflorescence of individualism in Renaissance Italy was due in the first place to the particular political circumstances of Italy from the thirteenth century.[120] In the first place, Burckhardt's Italians' sense of themselves as individuals involved a desire that their status and achievements were noteworthy, distinct from and elevated above any community. They sought recognition for difference and excellence. They did not ask to be

---

[116] Stone, *Family*, 151.   [117] Stachniewski, *The Persecutory Imagination*.
[118] Stone, *Family*, 152.   [119] Burckhardt, *Civilization*, 98–119.   [120] *Ibid.*, 98.

recognized for their unique interiority. The individualism of the Italian Renaissance did not assign a high value to self-scrutiny. The ideal of the *uomo universale*, represented, for instance, by Dante, was outwards facing. It was the aspiration to encompass the whole human and natural universe. Equally important, according to Burckhardt, were praise and fame. So, on Burckhardt's reading, Renaissance Italy became obsessed by a cult of celebrity.[121] The obverse of this desire for recognition was not a rich inwardness, but an equally status-obsessed culture of ridicule and wit.

The relation of individualism, self-consciousness, and melancholia that I am proposing is expressed in Figure 4.1. Melancholia, I contend, only occurs with any frequency within those Western traditions that have assigned intellectual or spiritual value to self-consciousness. For diagnoses of melancholia to be commonly made, there must be a cultural environment in which self-consciousness is highly valued. To the extent that individualism and self-consciousness overlap – and they do overlap to a considerable degree, but by no means completely – melancholia can also be found with individualistic cultures. But melancholic self-consciousness without individualism is entirely possible: witness Calvinism and Pietism. By the same token, melancholic individualism outside a culture that assigns high value to self-consciousness is found only rarely.

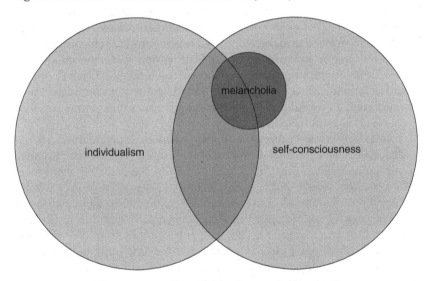

Figure 4.1 Melancholia, individualism, and self-consciousness.

---

[121] On individualism in Ancient Greece, compare Jacob Burckhardt, *The Greeks and Greek Civilization* (New York: St Martin's Press, 1998), 320–2: again desire for fame seems to have been the mainspring.

10   Confirmations and disconfirmations

The key advantage of the self-consciousness model is its empirical 'fit'. Where self-consciousness is found, there too melancholia is found; and where melancholia is found, we will find it in cultures that assign high value to self-consciousness. The self-consciousness model covers a wide area of the Western tradition from fifth-century BC Greece onwards. By contrast, the individualism models of Burckhardt, Weber, Tawney, Mauss, Morris, and Taylor are located in specific historical circumstances, notably Italian political institutions (Burckhardt), northern European capitalism (Weber and Tawney), or eleventh-century Augustinian Christianity (Morris), or in quite narrowly defined philosophical traditions: Stoicism (Mauss) or the line of descent from Plato through Augustine to Descartes (Taylor). The limitations of these models are nowhere more striking than in the case of Ancient Greece and Rome. The medical theory of melancholia was formulated not later than the fifth century BC, and it soon spilled over from medical writings into literary culture, and presumably was in fairly widespread use in society at large, especially in Athens.[122] Melancholia continued to be discussed through Graeco-Roman antiquity and into the Islamic Middle Ages. These facts are no less in need of explanation than the supposed epidemic of melancholia in early modern Europe. Explanations that draw on politically or socio-economically grounded individualism (Burckhardt, Weber, and Tawney) have no force here. The self-consciousness model is a better fit.

Hippocratic medicine placed a strong emphasis on autopsy: symptoms must be observed and studied at first hand, dispassionately and meticulously. A diagnosis of melancholia required careful observation of mental and emotional behaviour. Close observation of behaviour was a feature of Greek culture in general. Pre-classical and classical Greek literature, from Homer to Euripides and beyond, contains ample evidence of this. It is surely no coincidence that melancholia originated in a cultural environment that placed such a high value on knowing the self. In other words, in classical Greece just as in early modern Europe, melancholia was supported by a culture that placed a high value on self-consciousness. That is not to say that Ancient Greek self-consciousness was the same as early modern European self-consciousness, though one can reasonably argue that the differences between them have been exaggerated. For instance, Taylor argues that Ancient Greek melancholia and early modern

---

[122] *Melancholia* and cognates appear in the philosophers Plato and Aristotle, the tragedian Sophocles, the orator Demosthenes, and the comedians Aristophanes, Menander, and Alexis. See the relevant articles in Henry George Liddell and Robert Scott, *A Greek-English Lexicon* (Oxford University Press, 1996).

melancholia were fundamentally different. For the Greeks, melancholia resided in the black bile; for the early moderns, melancholia was part of the self.[123] The evidence presented in Chapters 1 and 2 suggests otherwise. The most consistently recorded symptoms of Graeco-Roman melancholia, and the symptoms that Galen viewed as melancholia's nosological core, were fear and sadness.

Taylor's history of the 'discovery of the self' involves denying the Ancient Greeks a developed sense of selfhood. The argument is in part a linguistic one. Ancient Greek had no stable word for 'self'.[124] (One might argue *au contraire* that Ancient Greek had a wide repertoire of means of expressing the idea of selfhood, precisely because the prefix *auto-* was so extensively and variously applicable.) Consequently Ancient Greek and early modern concepts of self-knowledge, while superficially similar, are quite different.[125] There was certainly nothing in Ancient Greece like the continuous and unabated introspection found in some post-Reformation Christianity. Often Greek self-knowledge was focused on external relations, such as one's relation to the gods or society. But *pace* Taylor, it could and frequently did turn inwards. The injunction 'know thyself' (*gnōthi seauton*) was inscribed in the forecourt of the temple of Apollo at Delphi. 'Know thyself' was not only a religious injunction, a mark of obedience to the healer god Apollo. It appears repeatedly in Plato's writings, most often spoken by the character of Socrates. Evidently, Plato thought it an important philosophical maxim.[126] In this secular and very much inwardly directed form, the maxim coheres with another maxim of Socrates: 'the unexamined life is not worth living'.[127] And here the bond linking ancient and modern self-consciousness is deep and strong. Ancient Greek self-consciousness was rediscovered and reinterpreted in the early modern period. 'Know thyself' was an inspiration for some cases of self-consciousness that now strike us as typically early modern, from John Davies's 1599 poem 'Nosce teipsum' to Karl Philipp Moritz's project of a psychological journal, *Gnōthi sauton: Magazine for Empirical Psychology*, in the 1780s. And as Udo Thiel and Victor Caston have argued, significant elements of the early modern philosophical debate on consciousness were pre-empted by Plato and Aristotle.[128] From this perspective, Taylor's insistence of differentiating between Ancient Greek and early modern notions of self-consciousness look not a little like the

---

[123] Taylor, *Sources*, 188–9.   [124] *Ibid.*, 176.   [125] *Ibid.*
[126] See Plato, *Charmides*, 164d; *Protagoras*, 343b; *Phaedrus*, 229e; *Philebus*, 48c; *Laws*, II, 923a; *Alcibiades*, 124a, 129a, 132c.
[127] Plato, *Apology*, 38a.
[128] Thiel, *Early Modern Subject*, 11; Victor Caston, 'Aristotle on Consciousness', *Mind* 111 (2002), 751–815.

kind of Hegelian progressivism that equates modernity with sophistication and antiquity with naivety. As Bernard Williams has argued forcefully and, I think, correctly, in some respects the opposite may be true, both because we fail to do Ancient philosophy justice and because our supposedly superior modern notions of ethical agency may be much less well formed than we think they are:

What is certainly true is that, to a greater extent than the progressivist story claims, we rely on ideas that we share with the Greeks. In my view, that must be so, since the supposedly more developed conceptions [i.e. modern conceptions of moral consciousness] do not offer much to rely on. So far as such basic conceptions are concerned, the Greeks were on firm ground – often on firmer ground than ourselves.[129]

I am proposing, then, that the wide diffusion of melancholia in the West is best explained not by the rise of individualism but by the belief, found in large parts of Western history, in the virtue of self-consciousness. But what about periods of European history in which melancholia did not flourish? If both vectors were in place, the Hippocratic tradition of medicine and a belief in the virtue of self-consciousness, why did melancholia not flourish at all times and in all places from the fifth century BC onwards? In some periods Hippocratic medicine was lost to the West, notably during the Dark Ages between the fall of the Roman Empire and the appearance of Arabic learning in southern Italy and Spain in the eleventh century. Otherwise there would seem to be only one period in the West when, despite the availability of Hippocratic medicine, melancholia went into eclipse. As we noted in Chapter 1, during the Hellenistic era between Aristotle and the first century AD, there is virtually no mention of melancholia in the surviving texts. The simplest explanation for this is the lack of surviving medical literature from the period, indeed the relative lack of literature of any kind.[130] No complete medical texts survive from the period. We know the names of several Hellenistic medical writers, and we know something about what they wrote, thanks to discussions and quotations in later writers, especially Galen. These fragments provide no evidence that any of the Hellenistic physicians wrote about melancholia as a psychological disease. Galen quotes some substantial extracts from Diocles of Carystus, which treat melancholia as a disease of the stomach, and he criticizes another Hellenistic physician, Erasistratus, for failing to discuss melancholia.[131] A second factor might

[129] Bernard Williams, *Shame and Necessity* (Berkeley, CA: University of California Press, 1993), 8. Williams uses the term 'progressivist' (4).
[130] Vivian Nutton, *Ancient Medicine* (London: Routledge, 2004), 140.
[131] Jouanna, 'At the Roots of Melancholy', 242.

also help to explain this absence. Interest in the Hippocratic humoral system seems to have waned during the Hellenistic period.[132] This was partly to do with developments in medical theory. The empirical school, established in the third century BC by Serapion of Alexandria and Philinus of Cos, rejected the aetiological approach of Hippocrates, instead focusing solely on symptoms and cures. Cures were applied to symptoms, not to diseases. This may account for the absence of melancholia in medical writings by the empiricists.

We can only speculate about the reasons for the absence of melancholia from the non-medical literature of the Hellenistic period. One factor may have been the rise of Stoic and Epicurean philosophy. Neither of these schools was especially interested in melancholia.[133] Nor were they particularly interested in self-knowledge. The Socratic elenctic method of achieving self-knowledge by means of question and answer played no part in either school. The spirit of Stoicism and Epicureanism was dogmatic. Its goal was not to engage its students in a process of truth-finding, but to have them fully internalize true doctrine. The Stoics and Epicureans were certainly interested in medical psychology and psychopathology. Both schools presented their doctrine as a kind of medicine for the mind. Epicurus compared philosophy to medicine and the philosopher to a doctor.[134] This was also part of Stoic ethics.[135] The mind was to be restored to health by purging false beliefs. There had for some time been a tendency in Greek philosophy to see the good life in psychological terms. The virtuous man must by definition be free from severe emotional disturbance.

The Greek tendency to marry psychology and ethics had accelerated with Aristotle. His perspective on psychology was dominated by ethical concerns, in particular by his focus on self-control and the curbing of immoderate anger. Aristotle does comment on melancholia, which he reinterprets as a disorder characterized by irritability.[136] This accords with Aristotle's interest in anger – an emotional state that may be desirable in appropriate measure and in the appropriate circumstances. Accordingly, Aristotle has much more to say about pure anger itself than about melancholia. Melancholia was only one, relatively insignificant way in which

[132] Flashar, *Melancholie*, 73.
[133] Pigeaud has argued that Lucretius was a major figure in the philosophical discussion of melancholia ('*Prolégomènes*', 506). In fact, Lucretius does not refer to melancholia either by name or by implication.
[134] Voula Tsouna, 'Epicurean Therapeutic Strategies', *The Cambridge Companion to Epicureanism*, ed. James Warren (Cambridge University Press, 2009), 249–65 (at p. 249).
[135] Brad Inwood and Pierluigi Donini, 'Stoic Ethics', in *The Cambridge History of Hellenistic Philosophy*, ed. Keimpe Algra et al. (Cambridge University Press, 1999), 675–738 (at pp. 711–12).
[136] Aristotle, *Nicomachean Ethics*, VII, vii, 8.

psychological dispositions might impinge on ethical behaviour. The Hellenistic schools of philosophy took Aristotle's approach further. Whereas Aristotle thought that moderate degrees of anger were compatible with virtue, the Stoics and Epicureans believed that a man could become wise only by completely suppressing emotional disturbances. Epicurus was particularly extreme in this regard. His philosophy was designed to make men happy by eradicating powerful emotions, and this concern explains the peculiar approach that they took to psychopathology. This focused on specific emotional problems, notably fear (of the gods and death) and desire (for wealth and fame). In Epicurean teaching the source of all unhappiness was psychological disturbance (Greek *tarachos*),[137] specifically the fears and desires caused by false beliefs. Some of the traditional symptoms of melancholia reappeared here in new guise. For instance, Lucretius' notion of 'care' (*cura*) in *De rerum natura* comprises fear and uneasiness but places relatively little emphasis on sadness. The overlap between melancholia and *cura* suggests that, had the Epicureans been so inclined, they might have adapted melancholia to suit their own priorities, as Aristotle did. But Epicureanism was generally intolerant of traditional forms of thought. The element of despondency in melancholia may simply not have suited the Epicureans' ethical perspective on the emotions. They evidently had no use for it.

The self-consciousness model provides a handy explanation for the absence of melancholia from Epicureanism and Stoicism. Far from assigning a high value to self-consciousness, as Plato had done, these schools of philosophy were actively opposed to it. The Stoics did develop a novel notion of legal and political individuality. Marcel Mauss argued that Stoic selfhood was one of the stages leading to modern notions of the individual.[138] Thiel, by contrast, points out that Stoic notions of political and ethical personhood are very different from and had little impact on early modern reflections on the self.[139] The problem with Mauss's argument is that the Stoics, like the Epicureans, aimed to free people from their concern for or about the psychological dimension of selfhood or, if you like, self-consciousness. The mind was to be fully refocused on its relation to the external world (Epicureanism) or reason (Stoicism). A mind in tune with nature and reason would necessarily be healthy, according to Epicurean and Stoic doctrine. It is true that the Stoics were able to

---

[137] See, for example, Epicurus, *Letter to Herodotus*, 81.

[138] Marcel Mauss, 'A Category of the Human Mind: The Notion of Person; the Notion of Self', in Michael Carrithers, Steven Collins, and Steven Lukes (eds.), *The Category of the Person: Anthropology, Philosophy, History* (Cambridge University Press, 1985), 1–25 (at pp. 18–19).

[139] Thiel, *Early Modern Subject*, 14.

entertain the question of whether a wise man could become mad. But the answer was 'no'. At most he might suffer from 'delusions resulting from melancholia or delirium', but not a complete alteration of his mental state or mood.[140] Any such profound mental disturbance arising from ordinary physical pathology was ruled out by Epicurean and Stoic ethics.

In this sense, the Hellenistic period might provide a confirmation *ex negativo* of the self-consciousness theory of melancholia. In the absence of a key vector – that is, the belief that self-consciousness is a route to happiness or virtue – the diagnosis of melancholia seems not to occur with any frequency. The niche in which melancholia thrived was formed by the two chief vectors of Hippocratic-Galenic medicine and a culture of self-consciousness. The absence of both of these vectors in a given historical period should also mean the absence of melancholia and, subject to reservations concerning the lack of literature from the period, which make any such thesis speculative, this is what we seem to find in the Hellenistic period.

11   The politics of early modern melancholia

If individualism-based models of melancholia in the tradition of Burckhardt, Weber, and Tawney cannot account for melancholia as a whole, they do find strong support in one early modern tradition. Melancholics often had political grievances, and they expressed these grievances in a melancholy mode. Melancholia provided forms of thought, speech and behaviour for political opposition, or it lent that opposition added rhetorical force. In expressing their opposition in this way, melancholics defined and asserted themselves as individuals like Burckhardt's Renaissance Italians. But individualism is by no means the end of the story. Self-consciousness also played an important role in melancholy politics. Political melancholia was often staged or acted out in complicatedly self-conscious ways.

The idea of political melancholia might seem counter-intuitive. Political intervention is active. Melancholia, if it has any political significance, is a passive affliction, something suffered by subjects or victims of political power. In this spirit Shoshana Felman has argued that madness is 'the opposite of rebellion. Madness is the impasse confronting those whom cultural conditioning has deprived of the very means of protest or self-affirmation.'[141] If madness expresses impotence, its cognitive content

---

[140] Diogenes Laertius, 7, 118.
[141] Shoshana Felman, *What Does a Woman Want? Reading and Sexual Difference* (Baltimore, MD: Johns Hopkins University Press, 1993), 21.

will surely be largely irrelevant. Much like Felman, in his 1968 study *Melancholy and Society*, Wolf Lepenies interpreted eighteenth-century German melancholia as the sublimation of the bourgeoisie's political will. In an age of princely absolutism the German bourgeoisie had no access to political power. Its unused political energies were channelled instead into philosophy and literature, resulting in an 'enforced hypertrophy of the realm of reflection'.[142] Following a pernicious precedent set by Luther, Germans tended to think that spiritual freedom could be enjoyed quite separately from political and social freedom. One could be truly, spiritually free even under absolute tyranny. So by a perverse logic, disenfranchisement, the very inability to influence politics, became a spiritual virtue. According to Lepenies, the late eighteenth-century melancholy themes of solitude and communion with nature were little more than the aimless and empty products of this disenfranchised idealism.

In Lepenies's view melancholia is the spectral absence of meaningful politics. Melancholia seems to lack the traditional virtues of political action: engagement, urgency, rational debate, and a sense of community. The lack of these virtues is most readily attributable to the psychological disposition of the melancholic. Felman's point seems to be – and this is an eery reminder of Foucault – that madness equates to unreason. But what if melancholia is understood as an idea rather than a disposition? In his study of pessimistic political theory, Joshua Foa Dienstag distinguishes between a meaningless pessimistic *disposition* and a potentially meaningful pessimistic *spirit*. His aim is to recover a lost tradition of political pessimism. The core ideas of this tradition are that time is a burden, the course of history is ironic, freedom and happiness are incompatible, and human existence is absurd.[143] In distinguishing between a pessimistic disposition and a pessimistic spirit, the former meaningless and the latter potentially meaningful, Dienstag means to defend himself against the charge of psychologism. But the defence may be unnecessary. Some of the main exponents of pessimism in the early modern period – Montaigne, Hume, and Rousseau are prominent – were by their own admission melancholics. They were also heirs of the Graeco-Roman philosophical tradition, which had made no categorical distinction between philosophical virtue and psychological disposition. The first to make such a categorical distinction was Immanuel Kant in the 1780s, when he moved the discussion of temperament from ethics to anthropology. Before Kant it was generally

---

[142] Wolf Lepenies, *Melancholy and Society* (Cambridge, MA: Harvard University Press, 1992), 61.
[143] Dienstag, *Pessimism*, 19.

assumed that temperament could inform ethics. Philosophical pessimism nourished and was nourished by a melancholy disposition.

In the following sections, I consider some examples of political melancholia in early modern literature. From Elizabethan and Jacobean theatre to the German Storm and Stress, melancholics expressed political protest *as melancholics*. Their protests may not have amounted to fully joined-up or notably sophisticated political thinking. Melancholics tended not to formulate fully worked out political agendas. To expect them to would be to misunderstand the function of melancholia: it did the work of criticism, not the work of constructive programme-building. But it was politically active and meaningful nonetheless.

12   Saturnine rebels and malcontents

The Elizabethan and Jacobean melancholic drew his political identity from two traditions, the characterology and psychopathology of melancholia in ancient medical writings, and melancholia's connection with the god Saturn, which originated in ninth-century Arabian astrology.[144] The ancient medical literature endued the melancholic with a number of unpleasant traits that later writers would combine into a portrait of irritability, vengefulness, and paranoia. The Hippocratic *Epidemics* record that melancholics are irritable and restless, angry, and prone to agitation.[145] Early modern writers on melancholia turned this irritability into jealousy and envy. Timothie Bright described melancholics as 'envious, and jelous, apt to take occasions in the worst part'.[146] For Burton the melancholic character was 'angry, waspish, displeased with every thing, *suspitious of all*'.[147] The idea of melancholic suspicion came from Rufus: '[T]he beginning of melancholy is indicated by fear, anxiety, and suspicion aimed at one particular thing.'[148] The combination of suspicion and fixation on one idea made melancholics seem prone to paranoia. In his *Discourse on the Preservation of Sight* (1594), André du Laurens says that '[T]he melancholike party is evermore suspicious, if he sees three or foure talking together, he thinketh that it is of him ... for being alwaies in feare, he thinketh verely that one or other doth lie in wait for him, and that some doe purpose to slay him.'[149] So too Burton: 'Most part *they are afraid they are bewitched,*

---

[144] Klibansky *et al.*, *Saturn*, 127–33.
[145] See, for example, *Epidemics*, Book II, 7, 2: Hippocrates, *Opera*, ed. Hugo Kuehlewein (Leipzig: Teubner, 1894–1902), vol. I, 235, 4.
[146] Timothie Bright, quoted by Babb, *Elizabethan Malady*, 30.
[147] Burton, *Anatomy*, vol. I, 204.   [148] Rufus, *On Melancholy*, 37.
[149] André du Laurens, *A Discourse of the Preservation of the Sight: of Melancholike Diseases; of Rheumes, and of Old Age* (London: Kingston, 1599), 93–4.

possessed, or poisoned by their enimies, and sometimes they suspect their neerest friends.'[150] The tendency towards paranoia is compounded by the melancholic's natural intelligence (see Rufus) and intransigence. Constantinus Africanus had said that melancholics become 'rigid in their principles'.[151] In Sir Thomas Elyot's *Castel of Helthe* (1533), the melancholic is 'styffe in opinions'.[152]

The figure of Saturn provided a mythic exemplar of how this disposition might crystallize into political form, at the same time as adding a new wealth of detail to the iconography of melancholia. The Graeco-Roman myths of Saturn presented a highly contradictory picture.[153] On the one hand, traditional myths depicted the reign of Saturn as a golden age of wealth and peace. Saturn presided over agriculture, maritime trade, and just rule. On the other hand, he was identified with the Greek god Kronos, who had brutally castrated and overthrown his father Uranus. It was prophesied that Kronos' child would in due course overthrow him, and he plotted to prevent this by devouring his children. Having lost the Olympian succession struggle to Zeus, he was exiled 'beneath the earth and the barren sea' (so Homer), where he brooded in solitude.[154] The negative aspect of the mythic Saturn could be confirmed by reference to astrology. In astrology Saturn was an inauspicious planet, the negative to Jupiter's positive, and associated with the colour black and the heavy, 'earthy' element lead.

The disparate and contradictory elements of the tradition were first formed into a coherent narrative in Raoul Lefèvre's romance *The Recuyell of the Historyes of Troye* (c. 1464: it was translated and printed under this title by Caxton, probably in 1472–3, the first printed book in English).[155] Lefèvre traced Saturn's melancholia back to the prophecy of his overthrow. Faced with destruction, Saturn chose banishment into brooding melancholia.[156] But this did not halt his long, slow decline, for eventually he fully internalized the prophecy of his fall in the form of a paranoid fixation, which drove him into open rebellion against Jupiter.[157]

Several types of saturnine political melancholic populate the literature of Elizabethan and Jacobean England. One type is the 'malcontent' who

---

[150] Burton, *Anatomy*, vol. I, 386–7.
[151] Quoted in Carol Falvo Heffernan, *The Melancholy Muse: Chaucer, Shakespeare, and Early Medicine* (Pittsburgh, PA: Duquesne University Press, 1995), 18.
[152] Thomas Elyot, *The Castel of Helthe*, 2nd edn (London: Berthelet, 1539), 3.
[153] Klibansky *et al.*, *Saturn*, 134.   [154] Homer, *Iliad*, XIV, 204.
[155] Donald A. Beecher, 'From Myth to Narrative: Saturn in Lefevre and Caxton', in *Saturn from Antiquity to the Renaissance* (University of Toronto Italian Studies 8), ed. Massimo Ciavolella and Amilcare A. Iannucci (Ottawa: Dovehouse, 1992), 79–90 (at p. 81).
[156] Beecher, 'Myth to Narrative', 84.   [157] *Ibid.*, 86.

rails at his 'corrupted age' in the manner of the Roman satirist Juvenal, as updated in the *Satyres* of John Marston.[158] The characterology of melancholia with its angry irritability and suspicion made the melancholic's voice a natural one for oppositional satire, but in this form of melancholy politics the disagreeable traits of melancholia were replaced by analogous positive traits. The malcontent might be heterodox in religion or political opinions or even actively seditious.[159] Often, though, melancholia was motivated by more personal concerns. A particular source of discontent was that the melancholic's talents had not been recognized.[160] Just as Juvenal had argued in his Third Satire that true merit went unrewarded, so Marston has a melancholic character claim that advancement has gone to others, to 'undeserving dullards'.[161] It may be that the melancholic has excluded himself from advancement precisely by virtue of his own excellence, as Burton suggested: 'He that is *Saturninus*, shall never likely be preferred. That base fellowes are often advanced, undeserving *Gnatoe's*, and vitious parasites, whereas discreete, wise, vertuous and worthy men are neglected and unrewarded.'[162] The implication is that in order to achieve political preferment one must be ruthless and sycophantic. The virtuous melancholic is simply not equipped for success in this world.

Exclusion from advancement was not normally sufficient grounds for sedition, though it might form part of a larger picture in which the principal motivation was a desire for revenge. The melancholy Saturn's rebellion against Jupiter became a motif in the genre of the revenge tragedy. In several notable cases the avenging rebel's melancholia is put on. Hamlet adopts a melancholic 'antic disposition' while he delays taking revenge on Claudius for his father's murder. The guise of melancholia allows Hamlet to satirize the court, especially the pompous and foolish fixer Polonius. In Marston's *The Malcontent*, Duke Altofronto has been removed from power in a coup and banished from Genoa. He returns in the guise of Malevole, the malcontent of the play's title, to satirize the corruption of the new court. In this guise he undermines the usurper and the Machiavellian courtier Mendoza and wins back his throne and wife. *The Revenger's Tragedy* (probably by John Middleton or Cyril Tourneur) also features a character who adopts the melancholic pose to camouflage his vindictive plotting. Vindice's beloved has been raped by the duke's son. With his brother Hippolito, Vindice hatches an elaborate plan to destroy the dynasty, which involves him acting the role of a man made

---

[158] The words of the character Bruto in Marston's satires: quoted in Babb, *Elizabethan Malady*, 80.

[159] Babb, *Elizabethan Malady*, 81.   [160] *Ibid.*, 76.

[161] Marston quoted by Babb, *Elizabethan Malady*, 80.   [162] Burton, *Anatomy*, vol. I, 192.

melancholy by a twenty-one-year-long court case. In summary, Hamlet, Altofronto, and Vindice are all made melancholy by events, but they overlay this authentic melancholia with a secondary, artificial veneer of melancholia. This has two uses: it gives them liberty to speak the truth to power and enables them to pass as mad and therefore harmless. Given that melancholia was traditionally associated with rebels and malcontents, it might seem odd that it could also be used as a mask of harmlessness. Perhaps it is a mark of the melancholic's cunning and his opponents' relative naivety that he perceives the duality but they do not.

Taking vengeance on political usurpers, as Altofronto and Hamlet do, is not much different from demanding the restoration of 'natural rights', which in practice meant the privileges of nobles to exercise power in their domains and to restrain the monarch. A classic fictional exponent of natural rights is the 'lean and hungry' Cassius in *Julius Caesar*. Unlike the other characters we have been discussing, Cassius has no need to feign melancholia. His melancholia sits naturally on him and is of a piece with his saturnine hatred of Caesar's tyranny.[163] This makes him singularly dangerous, as Caesar realizes:

> I fear him not:
> Yet if my name were liable to fear,
> I do not know the man I should avoid
> So soon as that spare Cassius. He reads much;
> He is a great observer and he looks
> Quite through the deeds of men: he loves no plays,
> As thou dost, Antony; he hears no music;
> Seldom he smiles, and smiles in such a sort
> As if he mock'd himself and scorn'd his spirit
> That could be moved to smile at any thing.
> Such men as he be never at heart's ease
> Whiles they behold a greater than themselves,
> And therefore are they very dangerous.[164]

Cassius is a melancholic in the tradition of Rufus, a man of 'excellent spirit', ingenuity, and natural intelligence. He also has something of Burton's 'discreete, wise, vertuous and worthy' melancholic. Caesar points to Cassius's envy of his greatness, but the play makes it clear that Cassius is a shrewder politician than Caesar, for while Cassius plots, Caesar is too vain to take precautions against rebellion. And Cassius

---

[163] Thomas McAlindon, *Shakespeare's Tragic Cosmos* (Cambridge University Press, 1996), 79–80, argues that Cassius is not melancholic but choleric. But Cassius's death is diagnosed as melancholic by Messala: 'Mistrust of good success hath done this deed. / O hateful Error, Melancholy's child' (*Julius Caesar*, Act V, scene iii, lines 65–6).

[164] Shakespeare, *Julius Caesar*, Act I, scene ii, lines 200–11.

comes very close to success. Had Cassius not been so dependent on the charismatic but woolly minded Brutus, Mark Antony would not have had the opportunity to turn Rome against the tyrannicides. Caesar is right, however, in another sense. Cassius envies the political success of Caesar, a man less talented than himself but possessed of a better balance of qualities. Cassius' lack of balance, above all an extreme commitment to self-consciousness that prevents him from recognizing his own true worth ('as if he mock'd himself'), means that he can never seem open and ingenuous to others. And so we return to the question of the melancholic's lack of advancement. The Elizabethan and Jacobean malcontent may well be an agent of political change, but the change desired by melancholics is generally change in a conservative direction. Melancholics are too self-interested to be agents of progress.

13   Retreatism

Lepenies began his study of the socio-political meanings of melancholia by aligning melancholia with the deviant phenomenon of 'retreatism'.[165] According to the US sociologist Robert K. Merton, retreatists reject the dominant goals and methods of their society and refuse to contribute to its orderly functioning. They are not rebels; they do not attempt to disrupt or undo society. Nor are they outsiders who set themselves beyond social norms. Retreatists withdraw from society while remaining within it. They form a silent and disengaged opposition.[166]

Retreatism is helpful for understanding a phenomenon of late seventeenth- and early eighteenth-century literature, the vogue for melancholy 'retirement' poetry. This is a genre that advocates retirement from the cares of commerce and politics. Its two principal themes are antipathy to city life and praise of simple rural delights. Anne Finch's poem 'A Nocturnal Reverie' offers a double form of escape, into rural peace and night-time. Night is an escape from the 'Cares', 'Toils', and 'Clamours' of the day.[167] Friendly night is preferred to the hostile 'fierce light' of day (line 40). It replaces confusion with 'compos'dness' and 'Quiet' (lines 43–5). Even the animals of farm and field share in this pleasure, for at night they are spared the troublesome attentions of men. Now they can enjoy 'their shortliv'd Jubilee . . . / Which but endures, whilst Tyrant-*Man* do's sleep' (lines 37–8).

[165] Lepenies, *Melancholy and Society*, 4–9.
[166] Robert K. Merton, 'Social Structure and Anomie', *American Sociological Review* 3 (1938), 672–82.
[167] Anne Finch, 'A Nocturnal Reverie', *The Poems of Anne, Countess of Winchilsea*, ed. by Myra Reynolds (University of Chicago Press, 1903), 268–70, line 49.

For the animals, night offers respite from exploitation by man. For humans things are more complex, because their battle is as much with an internal as with an external enemy. The problem is consciousness itself. The quality of night is that it allows the mind to find peace and ends the struggle with melancholic fear and anger, 'the Elements of Rage'. It is a sort of Epicureanism, but reimagined as an escape from melancholia:

> In such a *Night* let Me abroad remain,
> Till Morning breaks, and All's confus'd again;
> Our Cares, our Toils, our Clamours are renew'd,
> Or Pleasures, seldom reach'd, again pursu'd.   (lines 47–50)

Behind this genre of poetry stands the Roman Epicurean poet Lucretius, who advocated retirement from business and politics (*negotium*) and a life of philosophical leisure (*otium*) in the garden of Epicurus. Lucretius insisted that only Epicurean doctrine could bring peace to a troubled mind. All other forms of therapy were futile, let alone attempting to outrun mental troubles by changing one's location. In a similar vein, though often without the dogmatic optimism of Lucretius, seventeenth- and eighteenth-century retirement poetry acknowledges the nearly invincible power of melancholia, which cannot be overcome by mental struggle. The enemy is within, a part of our consciousness; neither physic nor philosophy can drive it out. One answer is merely to surrender, as the opening lines of Finch's 'Ardelia to Melancholy' propose:

> At last, my old inveterate foe,
> No opposition shalt thou know.
> Since I by struggling, can obtain
> Nothing, but encrease of pain.[168]

Struggling against melancholia only serves to exacerbate the illness. We make our melancholia worse by turning inwards, because melancholia feeds on self-consciousness. As Rufus sagely advised, it would be better if the sufferer were not aware of the illness in the first place.

The mood of the pastoral idyll extended beyond literature. Epicurean retirement was part of the ancestry of another great fashion of the eighteenth century, the English landscape garden. Here too, in attempting to relieve melancholia, one might easily fall into the kind of self-consciousness that made melancholia worse, not better. The English garden cultivated an appearance of naturalness and informality, in contrast to the highly formal French gardens popular on the Continent. The garden was a place to escape

---

[168] Anne Finch, 'Ardelia to Melancholy', *The Poems of Anne, Countess of Winchilsea*, 15–16, lines 1–4.

business and politics. It was precisely the naturalness of the English garden, at least in comparison to the more formal French style, that offered the prospect of release from care. In creating 'natural' spaces that offered an escape from care, English gardens often presented a somewhat fatalistic aspect: more like Finch's nocturnal retreat than the determinedly dogmatic garden of Epicurus. As a result, escape into the garden might be no escape at all, for the garden itself is shot through with melancholia. Nature is saturated by an uneasy consciousness of self, with symbols of memory, loss, and longing, such as follies, mock-classical temples, ruins, hermits' caves, and shrines to favourite dead dogs. (A grotto in the gardens of Rousham House near Oxford contains the inscription: 'In Front of this Stone lie the Remains of Ringwood an otter-hound of extraordinary Sagacity'.) In some cases the imagery of death was given a specific historical connection. One of the favourite tropes of the landscape garden was Elysium, home of the virtuous dead. William Kent, designer of the gardens at Rousham, constructed an Elysian Fields in the great gardens at Stowe. In this space alongside the familiar symbols of memory, loss, and melancholia, such as fallen tree trunks overgrown with ivy, were monuments to the virtuous dead of Britain and Ancient Greece. After Stowe's owner, Viscount Cobham, was expelled from Walpole's ministry and retired from politics in 1733, the Elysian Fields began to acquire a flavour of opposition to the Walpole government. In his 'Temple of British Worthies', Cobham erected busts of oppositional figures: Milton, John Hampden, and Sir John Barnard. The Greeks commemorated in Stowe's Temple of Ancient Virtue, notably Socrates, could also be interpreted as victims of state oppression.[169]

In the literature of sensibility, beginning around 1730, melancholia combines retreatism with oppositional politics, both in the specific political sense of Cobham's Stowe and in a broader Weberian economic sense. These political and economic meanings come to the fore in three closely related works from around 1770, Oliver Goldsmith's poem 'The Deserted Village' (1770), and the novels *The Man of Feeling* (1771) by Henry MacKenzie and Goethe's *The Sorrows of Young Werther* (1774). Alienation from economic progress can be felt in all three works. Britain's runaway economic growth upset traditional patterns of wealth distribution, and because it was grounded in the colonial trade, many Britons experienced it as distant and foreign. Although the German lands had no colonies to speak of, the European Atlantic nations' colonial enterprise, and slavery in particularly, was much criticized in Germany – for instance, by Goethe's

---

[169] Tim Richardson, *The Arcadian Friends: Inventing the English Landscape Garden* (London: Bantam, 2008), 306–28.

friend Herder. In all three works the same topos appears. The reader is given a tour of the town or village where the main figure of the work was born. We are shown what had once been a village schoolhouse, but has since been overtaken by economic progress. The schoolhouse has symbolic value because of its association with the Rousseauian theme of childhood. It represents an innocent past, before the advent of the adult world of commerce.[170] In Goldsmith's poem the schoolhouse has been abandoned because the land on which the 'sweet smiling village' stood has been bought up and 'enclosed' into a single property. The ostensible subject of the poem is the enclosure of common land and the consequent destruction of traditional ways of life:

> Thy sports are fled, and all thy charms withdrawn;
> Amidst thy bowers the tyrant's hand is seen,
> And desolation saddens all thy green:
> One only master grasps the whole domain.[171]

The process of enclosure and the destruction of the rural economy is driven by grasping capitalism: 'Ill fares the land, to hast'ning ills a prey, / Where wealth accumulates, and men decay' (lines 51–2). The poem's dominant mood is a melancholy sense of loss. The peasantry and the virtuous simplicity of their lives can never be replaced, now that the soulless forces of economic progress have been unleashed: 'times are alter'd; trade's unfeeling train / Usurp the land and dispossess the swain' (lines 63–4). The poem leads us through the site of the now deserted village. The spot on which the schoolhouse had stood is marked only by wild vegetation, 'blossom'd furze unprofitably gay' (line 194), which symbolically conveys the memory of a time when things with no economic value ('unprofitably') could survive.

MacKenzie's *The Man of Feeling* begins with a preface that explains how the text has survived.[172] The novel's 'editor' is out hunting with a fat, lazy cleric. The land they are on happens to be an 'inclosure' belonging to large 'melancholy' house, and the pursuit of game turns out to be futile, though the editor is compensated by the discovery of an interesting manuscript. His companion the cleric has been using some scraps of paper as gun wadding. These broken fragments contain the story of Harley, the eponymous man of feeling. The editor takes the shreds of Harley's story from the unfeeling cleric and so rescues them from destruction. The condition of the manuscript echoes the story of Harley's life. The text in fragments is a melancholy embodiment of a melancholy life.

---

[170] Barker-Benfield, *Culture of Sensibility*, 223.
[171] *Collected Works of Oliver Goldsmith*, ed. Arther Friedman, 5 vols. (Oxford University Press, 1966), vol. IV, 287–304, lines 36–9.
[172] Henry MacKenzie, *The Man of Feeling* (Oxford University Press, 2001), 3–5.

The novel operates with the familiar set of contrasts between sensibility and rationality, tradition and progress, failure and success, and it has a similar political thrust to Goldsmith's poem. The contrast between the evil city and virtuous country is made very clear. Harley is sent to London to pursue a legal claim for the lease of some land, and his experience of the city disillusions him. Returning home he meets the old farmer Edwards returning from the colonies, having been press-ganged into military service. Edwards and Harley lament the destruction of the old schoolhouse by the local squire, presumably the man who had the land enclosed. Like Goldsmith's village, poor Edwards has been ruined by colonialism, though his story illustrates a different dimension of the colonial enterprise. While in military service in the East Indies, he helped an innocent old Indian prisoner to escape. For his pains Edwards was court-martialled and expelled into the wilderness to face almost certain death, only to be saved in turn by the Indian. Critics have commented on the naivety of Edwards's story, which seems to suggest that the forces of colonialism could be opposed by acts of individual charity.[173] Through its admittedly simple narrative of one good turn provoking another, the novel makes a wider point. The largely impersonal forces of colonialism undermine moral values, but cannot completely extirpate them. 'The Deserted Village' also ends with an attack on colonial trade. The people of the destroyed village, 'a melancholy band' (line 401), are imagined queuing up at a port, as they wait to be shipped off to the colonies: 'to distant climes, a dreary scene, / Where half the convex world intrudes between, / Through torrid tracts with fainting steps they go' (lines 341–3). Goldsmith goes further than MacKenzie. Colonial trade is motivated by a desire for luxury that undermines society, and this is contrasted with solid traditional virtues: 'O Luxury!. . . / Kingdoms, by thee, to sickly greatness grown, / Boast of a florid vigour not their own' (lines 385–90). Cheyne had famously attributed the 'English Malady' to the physiological effects of luxury. *The Man of Feeling* and 'The Deserted Village' represent the melancholy effects of colonial trade in social and moral terms. These are (among other things) political statements; they use melancholia to diagnose a social ill. And they are, of course, fictional creations actively willed into being by their authors. Here melancholia evidently is not 'the impasse confronting those whom cultural conditioning has deprived of the very means of protest or self-affirmation' (Felman).[174]

---

[173] For instance, Stephen Bending and Stephen Bygrave, 'Introduction', in MacKenzie, *The Man of Feeling*, xvi–xvii.

[174] Felman, *What Does a Woman Want?*, 21.

Nor does Goethe's contemporaneous epistolary novel *The Sorrows of Young Werther* support Lepenies's view that German melancholia was the sublimation of the bourgeoisie's political will.[175] To be sure, political circumstances were different in Germany, and the opportunities for engagement in politics for a young bourgeois like Werther were very limited, as Lepenies rightly points out. But the most significant difference between the worlds of Goethe's and MacKenzie's novels is that although Goethe's generation were alert to the damage done by colonial trade, the chief focus of their anger was economic and political policies at home, notably the style of enlightened absolutist government that sought to reform society and the economy from above by concentrating political power in the princely courts. Like Harley, Werther is sent away to sort out some family legal business, though his departure from home also provides a welcome escape from a knotty romantic entanglement. Werther's first letter famously begins with the sentence: 'How happy I am to be away!'[176] Changing his location cannot change his melancholy temperament. Werther promptly falls in love with the beautiful, homely, but unavailable Lotte, and adds a dose of love melancholia to his already melancholy condition. Prescribed an activity cure for his melancholia, Werther takes up a post at a princely court. (Here life imitated art: Goethe would do the same the year after his novel was published, moving to the small Duchy of Sachsen-Weimar-Eisenach to work as the duke's mentor.) However, being a commoner, he finds himself excluded from the court's social life, and he resigns. After this failure he undertakes a symbol-laden return to his birthplace. At this point we encounter the familiar topos of the school-room that has been repurposed by the modern economy. Werther resents the changes wrought by progress in his hometown: 'I approached the town, saluting all the old, familiar bowers in the gardens and disliking the new ones, and disliking all the other changes that had been made as well.' We expect the same sentimental response to the old schoolhouse as we saw in Goldsmith and MacKenzie, but Werther gives us something very different. As he remembers his schooldays, memories of the horror of punishment and incarceration come flooding back to him: 'all the rest-lessness and tears, the heaviness of heart and the mortal fear I endured in that hole'.[177] *Werther* is an altogether more powerful work than 'The Deserted Village' or *The Man of Feeling*. A portrait of melancholy interiority unmatched perhaps since *Hamlet*, it represents the destructive forces of modernity at work on the hero's psyche. But *Werther* stands on the threshold of romanticism, and Werther's collapse into suicide is a kind

---

[175] Lepenies, *Melancholy and Society*, 61.   [176] Goethe, *Werther*, 25.   [177] *Ibid.*, 85–6.

of psychological Gothic, full of violent crises, hurtful recriminations, and help-seeking self-harm. Werther is alienated on many levels. At the same time his voice has a powerful authenticity, not least thanks to the style in which Goethe composed the novel. A non-standard German marked by regionalisms and archaisms, the novel's language is itself an act of nostalgic resistance against centralizing and modernizing tendencies in language reform. The power of the voice is then fractured by the book's form, for this is the first-ever one-sided epistolary novel. The main body of the novel consists of Werther's letters to his friend Wilhelm, but we are not given any of Wilhelm's replies. Werther's is a solitary voice in a vacuum.

14   Melancholy revolutions

The German Storm and Stress movement, with Goethe as its leading exponent, was both more vehement and more inventive in its forms of expression than anything in English literature of the period. Confused and frustrated though its politics undoubtedly was, it gives the lie to the idea that eighteenth-century melancholia was politically passive. Several Storm and Stress plays reprised the figure of the baroque malcontent, and served up a similar cocktail of revenge and political discontent. In the wake of American independence, young German authors were becoming more strident and confident. In Schiller's rebellious 1780 drama *The Robbers*, the hero Karl Moor is conceived as a latter-day melancholy Robin Hood, fighting injustice, corruption, and the abuse of power with an angry and weary heart.[178] The traditional revenge motif of the melancholy malcontent is also present. Karl sets out to avenge himself against a father who he erroneously believes to have disinherited him. In fact, Karl has been deceived by his similarly melancholy and malcontent younger brother Franz, who plans to drive a wedge between Karl and their father and so steal Karl's birthright. Both Karl and Franz are rebels. The play traces their different rebellions through parallel plots. Where Karl rebels against what he believes to be the abuse of power, Franz rebels against nature for having made him the ugly, uncharismatic second son. As with the malcontents of Jacobean drama, his complaint boils down to frustration at his lack of advancement and the world's failure to recognize his true genius. He formulates his rebellion in a positively Nietzschean revaluation of values. Morality, he says, is merely a ruse to pacify the gullible and should not hinder a genius like himself from self-realization. One of the play's parallel plots traces Karl's progressive disenchantment with his

---

[178] Friedrich Schiller, *The Robbers*, in Schiller, *The Robbers and Wallenstein*, trans. F. J. Lamport (Harmondsworth: Penguin, 1979).

revolutionary project because of its cost in human lives. The other plot follows Franz's descent into paranoid madness. This overarching move-ment creates space for violent swings between humanity and inhumanity, philanthropy and misanthropy. The play betrays a horrified fascination with human unpredictability. In rejecting human feeling and morality, Franz embarks on a rationalistic denial of his own emotions, but he ends up their victim. He discovers that power for its own sake empties the world of meaning. The moral vacuum he creates fills up with his own paranoid and suicidal fears.

After the traumatic execution of Louis XVI and the Terror, there was a general literary retrenchment across Europe, and the figure of the revolutionary malcontent took on more sombre tones. Schiller's tragic trilogy *Wallenstein* (1799), a drama as subtle in thought as it is epic in scale, reimagines the fate of the great Imperial general of the Thirty Years' War. In selecting his subject, Schiller knew that the historical Wallenstein had long been recognized as a melancholic, and he entan-gles his own Wallenstein in the complications and confusions of Renaissance Neoplatonic melancholia. A thoroughly saturnine figure, Wallenstein is misled by erroneous astrological advice into believing that he was actually born under the sign of the joyful Jupiter. Astrology also leads him to temporize like Hamlet, when in fact resolute action is required. In a decisive scene his subordinate Illo begs Wallenstein to act. Wallenstein replies with a passionate but strangely oblique speech rich in occult iconography. Illo, he implausibly claims, is a schemer like the 'subterranean god' Saturn:

> You know no better than you speak. How often
> Have I explained it to you! Jupiter,
> Bright-shining god, was set when you were born;
> These secrets are beyond your understanding.
> In earth to burrow is your place, blind like
> That subterranean god who lit your way
> Into this life with grey and leaden beams.
> Common and earthly things you may perceive,
> May shrewdly see the links that lie at hand;
> In this I trust you and believe your words.
> But what in mystery is woven, what
> Great secrets grown and shaped in Nature's depths –
> The spirit ladder, from this world of dust
> Ascending by a thousand rungs to reach
> The stars, and trod by countless heavenly powers
> Pursuing up and down their busy ways –
> The circles within circles, that draw close
> And closer yet upon the focal sun –

> These things the unclouded eye alone can see
> Of Jupiter's fair children, born in light.[179]

The irony of this speech is that Wallenstein is far from being one of 'Jupiter's fair children'. He, not Illo, is the saturnine schemer. Indeed, his superstitious belief in astrology symbolizes Wallenstein's melancholic infirmity. The longer he is misguided by astrology, the more passive he becomes and the more he succumbs to a crippling and fatal, Hamlet like procrastination. He fails to act on the secret negotiations he has entered into with the Swedish enemy, perhaps because he cannot decide what his aim is or cannot bring himself to admit it. Does he want peace for the empire? Or revenge on the emperor for relieving him of his command at Regensburg some years earlier? Or does he want the crown of Bohemia for himself and a royal husband for his daughter? In Wallenstein, Schiller reimagines the melancholy malcontent for a post-revolutionary age, as a mixture of political idealism, dark revenge, and naked self-advancement.

15   Melancholia, society, and self-consciousness

What does this historical and literary material tell us about the relation between melancholia and social status? While there is some evidence that modern capitalism might have exposed some of its main beneficiaries to melancholia, monocausal explanations are clearly insufficient. There is ample historical evidence that people who neither aspired to nor accumulated wealth suffered from profound melancholia. Indeed, considering the full range of evidence it would be hard to resist Opler and Small's conclusion that different negative social experiences can create different ways of being depressed. The depressed rich and the depressed poor are both depressed, only in different ways.[180] This should neither surprise nor trouble us. In this chapter's early sections we saw that different geographically determined life experiences could create different ways of being melancholy, as in the religious melancholia of the New England Puritans and the nostalgia of Swiss mercenaries. In principle, there is no reason why the same argument that applies to geographical niches should not apply to social niches. Different social niches bring different life experience and give rise to different ways of being melancholy. It is simply a matter of extending the theory of culture-bound syndromes to the social world.

---

[179] Schiller, *The Piccolomini*, lines 966–85, in Schiller, *The Robbers and Wallenstein*, 254.
[180] Opler and Small, 'Cultural Variables'.

From its beginnings melancholia was thought to afflict people according to their circumstances, whether through the six 'non-naturals' that worried physicians in the Hippocratic and Galenic tradition, or through the social and political troubles identified in many modern texts. The content of people's melancholy cognitions usually corresponded fairly closely to the causes of their melancholia. Melancholics were generally quite explicit about what was wrong with them and what they thought had caused it. Contrary to Freud's view that people's conscious thoughts usually bear no obvious relation to the dynamics of their mental illness, and that to uncover the latter considerable skilled work is required by the psychoanalyst, we could also say that melancholics were often well informed about what ailed them, or at least were quite good at identifying the approximate site of the problem.

This brings us to the question of causation. Do social problems cause melancholia, or does melancholia cause social problems? Causation in a strict medical sense, as in the sense in which cancer cells cause malignant tumours, will be very difficult to establish for something as complex and multicausal as melancholia. When I said that in many modern texts melancholia is a response to social and political circumstances, I meant that the response is processed through thoughts and feelings. In mental disorders of this kind, different causal factors typically combine into complex wholes and form self-perpetuating feedback loops. Melancholy affect may give rise to melancholy cognitions, but the cognitions can in turn cause the affective symptoms to worsen, and so on.

This raises another question: how much of the cognitive content of melancholia is just performance of a role that seems attractive or provides relief to the melancholic? Plenty of evidence exists for this kind of thing. Melancholia really was a fashionable disease, a disease whose modes of expression one might adopt because those very modes of expression – the behaviour, the clothes, the metaphors – seemed to fit and perhaps even gave some relief. The cognitive behaviour of melancholics contains a high degree of self-consciousness. Indeed, melancholia in its psychologically florid form can exist only because the West has developed a culture of self-consciousness which it esteems highly and considers part of its birthright. The ruminations on selfhood in *Hamlet*, *Werther*, and *Wallenstein* testify to that intimate bond between melancholia and self-consciousness.

5   The telescope of truth

1   Mental disorders and creativity

Early modern writers took a variety of positions on the politics of the melancholy malcontent, from Marston's cynical but noble Altofronto to Schiller's hesitant, clay-footed Wallenstein. All agreed though on the malcontent's potential brilliance as a politician, even though that potential was often unrealized, whether because the political goal was misguided, the execution was frustrated by prevarication, or the outcome was marred by tragic violence. Subject to certain qualifications, then, in these works there seems to be a fairly consistent link between melancholia and exceptional intelligence, of a kind that we have seen in Rufus ('those of subtle mind and great insight easily fall prey to melancholia') and the pseudo-Aristotelian *Problems* XXX/1 with its famous beginning: 'Why is it that all men who have become outstanding in philosophy, statesmanship, poetry or the arts are melancholic?'[1]

Why indeed? For literary malcontents an answer immediately suggests itself. The literary malcontent embodies a certain style and tradition of poetic self-presentation. Poets gravitated towards the idea of the melancholy genius as a way of imagining and presenting themselves. The tradition of the melancholy poet had the sanction of antiquity and of Aristotle's name. The author of *Problems* XXX/1 had claimed that among melancholics were to be counted 'most of those who have handled poetry'. Inspired by this text, the writers of the Italian Renaissance, notably Petrarch, Ficino, and Tasso, defined themselves as melancholics. The Renaissance tradition of the melancholy writer added the Platonic idea of divine poetic madness to *Problems* XXX/1, so imbuing it with an extra philosophical force that combined well with the Platonic nuances already contained in the *Problems*. However, the account of genius in *Problems* XXX/1 is physiological, not psychological. The grand claim that all men of genius have been melancholics is not backed up with a

[1] Aristotle, *Problems* II, 154.

152

reasoned psychological case explaining why it should be so. Instead we find a not altogether coherent account of the heating of the bile and its effects on behaviour. Despite this lack of a psychological argument, *Problems* XXX/1 inspired a great number of representations and self-representations of melancholy artists. In the early modern period the figure of the melancholy artist was something of a commonplace. And as for poets, so for their themes: since the Renaissance a disproportionate quantity of literature (and art and music) has taken melancholia as its theme.

Problems XXX/1 is often quoted in modern attempts to link artistic creativity and mental illness, though more for its quaintness and antiquity than for any explanatory force it might have.[2] But aside from the historical legacy of the *Problems*, is there any natural connection between melancholia and artistic creativity? Psychiatry has been fascinated by genius since the middle of the nineteenth century.[3] Interest peaked in the 1990s with the publication of Kay Jamison's *Touched with Fire* (1994) and Arnold Ludwig's *The Price of Greatness* (1995). Both analysed the biographies of (dead) eminent creative people. Jamison focused on writers, artists, and composers and singled out Byron for a special case study. Ludwig looked more broadly at eminent members of the creative and other professions. Both adopted the same approach of using the written record – biographies or autobiographies or creative writing – to diagnose their subjects' declared or undeclared mental illness. The diagnosis was retrospective, since the subjects were dead, some of them long dead. Jamison investigated correlations between her subjects' documented mental state and certain statistically significant features of bipolar disorder such as changes in cognitive behaviour, seasonal variations in occurrence, and heritability. Ludwig conducted a similar analysis of the statistical prevalence of family problems, behavioural attributes, and sexual orientation. They reached broadly the same conclusion: that a link of some kind exists between creativity and bipolar disorder (Jamison) or between creativity and a range of depressive disorders (Ludwig).

The hypothesis of a link between artistic creativity and bipolar disorder is attractive, but how would we test it? The Jamison–Ludwig approach of retrospective diagnosis is fraught with problems, not least because

[2] See, for example, Kay Redfield Jamison, *Touched with Fire: Manic-Depressive Illness and the Artistic Temperament* (New York: Free Press, 1993), 51.
[3] Jacques-Joseph Moreau, *La Psychologie morbide dans ses rapports avec la philosophie de l'histoire, ou De l'influence des névropathies sur le dynamisme intellectuel* (Paris: Masson, 1859); César Lombros [Cesare Lombroso], *L'Homme de génie* (Paris: Schleicher, 1889); Paul Julius Möbius, 'Über das Studium der Talente', *Zeitschrift für Hypnotismus* 10 (1902), 66–74.

psychiatric nosological categories have changed significantly over even recent time. Some of what counted as mental illness in the past does not now and vice versa. And behaviours that have consistently counted as mental illness over hundreds of years are theorized quite differently now from how they were theorized in the past. One might take the view that theoretical change does not matter. Indeed, one might argue that theoretical change is precisely the reason we need diagnose retrospectively. In the historical past, symptoms may have been diagnosed incorrectly. Using modern categories, we can correct the historical diagnoses. But there are several reasons why this will not do. Symptoms recorded in biography or autobiography cannot be incorporated unproblematically into a medical diagnosis. The reporting and collating of symptoms was not done to standards that would be acceptable now; most of the evidence, especially from fiction and biography, is anecdotal. But even symptoms recorded in a formal medical context are more or less unusable, as they cannot be teased apart in any unproblematic way from the theories that pertained at the time of diagnosis. After all, data determines theory, but theory also determines what data are relevant. Finally, the numbers of cases are so small and the evidence so patchy that dead poets could never constitute a statistically or methodologically valid sample. There is no empirical warrant for the retrodiagnosis of bipolar disorder in dead poets, and it is hard to see how there ever could be.

The conventional approach is to conduct fresh research using living subjects, and a good deal of work of this kind has been done recently. The field of creativity research is large and flourishing and extends across a number of subdisciplines of experimental psychology – social, organizational, cognitive, clinical, and child psychology.[4] Of special relevance to our discussion is the study of creativity from the perspective of personality and mood. There is some evidence that depressed or elevated mood affects creativity, although the evidence is contradictory. Some studies show that depressed mood enhances creativity; others the opposite. Further research in this area may yield more conclusive results, but even if it did, it would be hard to see how this research could answer the question addressed in the *Problems*: how does melancholia relate to artistic genius? The chief difficulty is the concept of creativity itself. Creativity researchers agree on a broad definition of their object. Creative thought is characterized by its fluency (the number of solutions to problems that a person can produce), its adaptability and flexibility (the range of types of

---

[4] For an overview, see Matthijs Baas, Carsten K. W. De Dreu, and Bernard A. Nijstad, 'A Meta-Analysis of 25 Years of Mood–Creativity Research: Hedonic Tone, Activation, or Regulatory Focus?', *Psychological Bulletin* 134 (2008), 779–806 (at p. 779).

problems that can be solved), and its originality (the innovative nature of the solutions).[5] However, there is little agreement on how to measure these elements.[6] Most experimental research employs small-scale problem-solving exercises, but this notion of creativity bears very little resemblance to the creative processes that produce major works of art. Problem-solving is far from being the sole defining feature of artistic creation. And creativity is only one element in artistic excellence. Formal craft and skill would also need to be measured, as would the subtlety and complexity of the works' cognitive content. Even where modern research has tried to measure actual artistic creativity – in a 1985 study participants were required to compose haikus that were then assessed for their originality[7] – these have been on too small a scale to confirm or disconfirm the sort of claims made by Jamison and Ludwig. In saying this I do not mean to disparage the haiku: my point is just that one can well imagine a person of otherwise average creativity getting lucky with one haiku. A more appropriate test would be haiku composition over an extended period, the whole career of a haiku poet. Some studies have tried to address this longitudinal problem by constructing samples that reflect a lifetime of creativity or intelligence. A study that followed a large sample of Swedish schoolchildren into adulthood found a high correlation between excellent academic achievement and a tendency to develop bipolar disorder in later life. It may be that the cognitive styles found in bipolar manic episodes (e.g. verbal inventiveness, mental stamina, highly emotional thinking) lend themselves to creative work. But the study also found that bipolar disorder was associated with very poor academic performance. Perhaps the cognitive styles found in bipolar disorder predispose students to perform either extremely well or extremely badly.[8] A further question is whether the tendency to develop bipolar disorder was a genetic predisposition (which would speak for Jamison's view) or perhaps a result of the peculiar stresses of being highly creative or intelligent (which would speak against it). In other words, does depression cause creativity or does creativity cause depression? A similar question was asked by the eighteenth-century French *philosophe* Helvétius concerning the relation between melancholia and intelligence. He concluded that highly intelligent people were melancholics because of their intelligence, not intelligent because of their melancholia: '[T]he most spiritual and

[5] Baas *et al.*, 'Meta-Analysis', 780–1.   [6] *Ibid.*, 780.
[7] T.M. Amabile, 'Motivation and Creativity: Effects of Motivational Orientation on Creative Writers', *Journal of Personality and Social Psychology* 48 (1985), 393–7.
[8] James H. MacCabe *et al.*, 'Excellent School Performance at Age 16 and Risk of Adult Bipolar Disorder: National Cohort Study', *British Journal of Psychology* 196 (2010), 109–15.

thoughtful people are, I know, often melancholics; however, they are not spiritual and thoughtful because they are melancholics, rather they are melancholics because they are thoughtful.'[9] The longitudinal data collected by Arnold Ludwig appear to contradict Helvétius by showing that mental illness sets in before *people* launch their creative careers, which might suggest that bipolar disorder is not a consequence of the stresses of intelligence or creativity.[10] But the issue cannot be settled quite so simply. After all, it may be that creative people suffer the depressogenic effects of being creative before actual creative activity begins. After all, some writers have to wait until later life to produce outstanding work or even to write at all, though their potential to do so was presumably present long before. One way to settle this issue and confirm or disconfirm the genetic thesis would be to examine the prevalence of bipolar disorder in the families of creative people. If the families of creative types show a higher-than-average incidence of bipolar disorder, it might indicate a genetic link between bipolar disorder and creativity. Jamison and Ludwig retrodiagnosed bipolar disorder and other affective disorders in the families of their subjects and claimed to find higher than normal levels of the disorder. A 1988 study complicated the picture by appearing to show that the healthy relatives of bipolar disorder sufferers enjoy higher levels of creativity than their bipolar relatives or those with no family history of mental illness at all. Perhaps the relatives of bipolar disorder patients had subclinical levels of hypomania, a state characterized by abnormally high but subpathological levels of mental activity.[11] This might be true more generally of the connection between mental illness and creativity. Some disorders, such as bipolar disorder, depression, anxiety, and even alcohol abuse, might be conducive to creativity at low levels, but unconducive at high levels.[12]

2   Depressive realism

The studies cited here contain a wealth of indications that psychopathology and creativity are somehow connected, but none of these studies are close to being conclusive. Where literature is concerned, measures of

---

[9] 'Les plus spirituels et les plus méditatifs sont quelquefois mélancoliques, je le sais: mais ils ne sont pas spirituels et méditatifs parcequ'ils sont mélancoliques, mais mélancoliques parcequ'ils sont méditatifs', Claude-Adrien Helvétius, *De l'Homme*, in Helvétius, *Œuvres* (Paris: Didot l'aîné, 1795), vol. VIII, 138–9.

[10] Arnold M. Ludwig, *The Price of Greatness: Resolving the Creativity and Madness Controversy* (New York: Guilford Press, 1995), 5.

[11] Ruth Richards *et al.*, 'Creativity in Manic-Depressives, Cyclothymes, Their Normal Relatives, and Control Subjects', *Journal of Abnormal Psychology* 1988 (97), 281–8.

[12] Ludwig, *Price*, 8.

creativity and intelligence are blunt instruments. While the hypothesis that bipolar disorder may be at least partly responsible for Byron's brilliance as a poet has a certain allure, it reduces something rich and complex to something rather simple-minded. If we are going to talk meaningfully and sensitively about the psychology of poetic creativity, we need to give a much fuller account of the conscious and unconscious processes involved in the creation of poetic meaning, and psychological research into creativity has not yet done so. For instance, this research has little to say about the cognitive content of literature. One area still to be explored is the connection between the content of melancholy writing and the cognitive psychology of depression. In entertaining this sort of research, I do not mean to suggest that studying the content of poetry is in any way adequate. All I mean is that it would go some way towards meeting the legitimate demands of a theory of literature. It would certainly be more sympathetic and less reductive than trying somehow to measure poetic creativity. It might also take advantage of recent work in the cognitive psychology of depression. The remainder of this chapter offers a tentative and admittedly only partial attempt to connect the cognitive psychology of depression with the literature of melancholia.

Since the 1970s, the cognitive psychology of depression has been a lively and controversial subject. Particular controversy has surrounded what has become known as the 'depressive realism' or 'sadder but wiser' hypothesis. Depressive realism was first posited in a study by Lauren Alloy and Lyn Abramson in 1979. In their first experiments Alloy and Abramson tried to measure the degree of control subjects thought they were exercising over a contingent situation. The subjects, half of whom were diagnosed with depression, the other half not, were placed in front of a box containing a green light which either would or would not light up after the subjects pressed one of two buttons. The boxes were all pre-programmed in different ways to be more or less responsive to the pressing of the button. The subjects were then asked to assess how much control they thought they had over the outcome. The results seemed to show that the depressed subjects formed more accurate assessments of the degree of control they were exercising than the non-depressed control group did. Alloy and Abramson followed this up with a study of the ways in which depressed students predicted their own examination results. This appeared to show that depressed students made more accurate predictions of their results than non-depressed students. The depressed students gave relatively accurate predictions of their grades; the non-depressed students tended to inflate or overestimate theirs.[13]

---

[13] Lauren B. Alloy and Lyn Y. Abramson, 'Depressive Realism: Four Theoretical Perspectives', in Lauren B. Alloy (ed.), *Cognitive Processes in Depression* (New York: Guilford Press, 1988), 223–65 (at p. 233).

The results of both studies threatened to overturn conventional wisdom. Previous theories of depressive cognition, notably Seligman's theory
of 'learned helplessness' and Beck's cognitive behavioural theory, had
assumed that depression was characterized by cognitive distortions.[14] If
you were depressed, you had a distortedly negative view of the world and
yourself. These cognitive distortions were one of the sources of your
depression. Healthy people, by contrast, would have a realistic picture of
the world. Good mental health was ensured by a process of continual and
successful 'reality checking'. By calibrating your assumptions against
reality, you could correct misconceptions and prevent yourself falling
victim to harmful delusions. (Of course, this always begged the question:
what is reality?)

According to these established theories of depressed cognition,
mentally healthy people assess reality more accurately than mentally
ill people. So what sense could be made of Alloy and Abramson's
depressive realism? In a subsequent paper Alloy and Abramson proposed a reversal of traditional assumptions. Whereas established models
assumed that it was depressed people who suffered from cognitive
biases, Alloy and Abramson now argued that healthy thinking was shot
through with biases:

> Depressed individuals may be suffering from the absence or breakdown of normal
> optimistic biases and distortions. Maladaptive symptoms of depression, such as
> low self-esteem, social skills deficits ... may be consequences, in part, of the
> absence of healthy personal illusions.[15]

So are healthy people generally more prone to cognitive illusions? The
work of Daniel Kahneman and Amos Tversky suggests that normal cognition is indeed shot through with illusions. Kahneman and Tversky have
argued that our normal cognitive functioning involves a number of short-
cuts or 'heuristics', which ease and accelerate the forming of judgements,
at the cost of reflecting reality accurately. For instance, we tend to assume
that the outcome of a causal process will have some resemblance to the
causal factors that generated it (the heuristic of 'representativeness'). Or
we will often assess a situation not in terms of its actual circumstances, but
in terms of whatever information about it happens to be close to hand or
uppermost in our minds ('availability'). And when we make rough and
ready arithmetical calculations, we tend to work from an initial or 'anchor'

---

[14] Martin E. P. Seligman, *Learned Helplessness: On Depression, Development, and Death* (San
Francisco: Freeman, 1975), and Aaron T. Beck, *Cognitive Therapy and the Emotional
Disorders* (Harmondsworth: Penguin, 1989).

[15] Alloy and Abramson, 'Depressive Realism', 257. See also Shelley E. Taylor and Jonathon
D. Brown, 'Illusion and Well-Being', *Psychological Bulletin* 103 (1988), 193–210.

value that may not be well computed ('anchoring').[16] Could it be that depressed people are less optimistic about the adequacy of these and other heuristics and so less prone to the cognitive illusions they generate?[17]

The study of cognitive illusions is a lively and contested field. On the one hand, the idea that 'rational' or healthy thought is shot through with cognitive distortions seems to be consistent with the depressive realism hypothesis.[18] Studies have shown that depressed people are less blind to negative aspects of their surroundings, whereas healthy people tend to ignore negative data.[19] Depressed people also tend to pay equal attention to both negative and positive feedback; non-depressed people tend to pay excessive attention to positive feedback.[20] But the depressive realism hypothesis has been criticized. Some researchers have been unable to replicate the depressive realism effects found by Alloy and Abramson.[21] Others have argued that depressive realism is an artefact of contrived experimental scenarios.[22] Some evidence suggests that depressed people exercise excessive rational control in trivial situations, but that in situations of more consequence the benefits of depressive realism

[16] Amos Tversky and Daniel Kahneman, 'Judgment Under Uncertainty: Heuristics and Biases', *Science* 185/4157 (1974), 1124–31.

[17] Benjamin M. Dykman *et al.*, 'Processing of Ambiguous and Unambiguous Feedback by Depressed and Nondepressed College Students: Schematic Biases and Their Implications for Depressive Realism', *Journal of Personal and Social Psychology* 56 (1989), 431–45 (at pp. 432–3).

[18] Sanford Golin, Francis Terrell, and Barbara Johnson, 'Depression and the Illusion of Control', *Journal of Abnormal Psychology* 86 (1977), 440–2; Sanford Golin *et al.*, 'The Illusion of Control Among Depressed Patients', *Journal of Abnormal Psychology* 88 (1979), 454–7; Robert C. Smolen, 'Expectancies, Mood, and Performance of Depressed and Nondepressed Psychiatric Inpatients on Chance and Skill Tasks', *Journal of Abnormal Psychology* 87 (1978), 91–101; C. S. Tang and J. W. Critelli, 'Depression and Judgment of Control: Impact of a Contingency on Accuracy', *Journal of Personality* 58 (1990), 717–27.

[19] R. E. Nelson and W. E. Craighead, 'Selective Recall of Positive and Negative Feedback, Self-Control Behaviors and Depression', *Journal of Abnormal Psychology* 86 (1977), 379–88.

[20] Lauren B. Alloy and Alan J. Lipman, 'Depression and Selection of Positive and Negative Social Feedback: Motivated Preference or Cognitive Balance?', *Journal of Abnormal Psychology* 101 (1992), 310–13.

[21] A sample of the critical literature: C. Randall Colvin and Jack Block, 'Do Positive Illusions Foster Mental Health? An Examination of the Taylor and Brown Formulation', *Psychological Bulletin* 116 (1994), 3–20; Keith S. Dobson and Dennis Pusch, 'A Test of the Depressive Realism Hypothesis in Clinically Depressed Subjects', *Cognitive Therapy and Research* 19 (1995), 179–94; Rachel M. Msetfi *et al.*, 'Depressive Realism and Outcome Density Bias in Contingency Judgments: The Effect of the Context and Intertrial Interval', *Journal of Experimental Psychology. General* 134 (2005), 10–22; Rachel M. Msetfi, Robin A. Murphy, and Jane Simpson, 'Depressive Realism and the Effect of Intertrial Interval on Judgements of Zero, Positive, and Negative Contingencies', *Quarterly Journal of Experimental Psychology* 60 (2007), 461–81.

[22] Lorraine G. Allan, Shepard Siegel, and Samuel Hannah, 'The Sad Truth About Depressive Realism', *Quarterly Journal of Experimental Psychology* 60 (2007), 482–95.

disappear.[23] Even assuming that depressive realism is real, it is not clear precisely what features of depressed cognition are responsible for it. Depressive realism shows some promise, but we would be wise not to get too excited about it just yet.

3   Melancholia as cultural content

Even if all the methodological caveats raised in the last two sections could be assuaged, we would still be faced by the seemingly impenetrable black box of the creative mind. Generations of scholars have been tempted by the siren song of *Problems* XXX/1, with its quaintly blithe assurance that all poets have been melancholics. But the fact is that psychology has very little to say about artistic creativity. There is an alternative, however. Instead of asking what it is in the psychology of melancholics that makes them good artists, we could ask why there is so much melancholy art. Why has melancholia been such a popular theme in Western culture? What is it about the cognitive content of melancholia – pessimism, nostalgia, self-doubt, anxiety – that makes it aesthetically useful or attractive? Formulated in this way, the question ceases to be psychological and becomes instead a question about the cultural history of psychological theory, and here the tradition of melancholia furnishes us with solid evidence. This is where the depressive realism hypothesis, for all the legitimate worries about its validity, might be helpful: by pointing us towards the sort of features of melancholy psychology that have tradition-ally been associated with special creative insight.

What I want to argue is that the depressive realism hypothesis is inter-esting for what it could tell us about depressive cognitive behaviour. If the depressive realism hypothesis is correct, melancholy cognition may have the power to cut through conventional illusions, to replace optimistic healthy illusions with a more compelling truth. If we transfer this idea to the cultural sphere, we might be able to argue that melancholy art has a special force, a capacity to move us from our conventional assumptions to a different and more compelling vision of reality. In other words, depres-sive realism might provide a way to understand the specific characteristics and qualities of melancholy art. Again I want to stress that this approach is quite different from the psychological approaches to creativity described in section 1 of this chapter. The argument is not that depressive realism explains the psychology of depressive creativity; this is not an attempt to

---

[23] Rosemary Pacini, Francisco Muir, and Seymour Epstein, 'Depressive Realism from the Perspective of Cognitive-Experiential Self-Theory', *Journal of Personality and Social Psychology* 74 (1998), 1056–68.

get inside the creative process. On the contrary, I want to use depressive realism to explain why the cognitive content of melancholy culture has been taken seriously in aesthetic terms. In some circumstances melancholics may believe that they make better judgements than non-melancholics. In a similar way, melancholy art may contain symptomatic (i.e. specifically melancholic) cognitive behaviours that turn out to be of particular artistic value. However, the depressive realism hypothesis is not an aesthetic theory. It cannot pretend to demonstrate the aesthetic quality of melancholy works of art. To show that melancholia makes great art would involve detailed critical engagement and interpretation, which would be well beyond the competence of the depressive realism hypothesis. Still, using depressive realism we can usefully address two issues here. First, we can try to explain the breadth of melancholia's cultural appeal. Why has melancholy art been so significant in the Western cultural tradition? Second, we can perhaps explain why melancholia has been such a force in high-concept aesthetics. Why have poets in particular tried to explain their practice with reference to melancholia? Ideally, we would look at music, the visual arts, and literature, but the first two are beyond my expertise, so in what follows I shall take only the briefest of glimpses at non-literary artistic production. Most of this chapter will be concerned with the history of literature in Western Europe. The aim will be to show how the cognitive contents of melancholia have fed into literary practice and programmatic aesthetic utterances.

In the history of Western music, melancholia has been much more common than the other three Galenic humours. Why should this be so? I suggest there are two reasons. First, whereas traditional medicine generally considered the four humours to be an ensemble, such that where one was discussed, the others would usually also appear, in the arts this ensemble treatment proved too unwieldy. It required the artist to create a work with a four-part structure, each element of which would illustrate one of the four humours. And we do indeed find examples of works of visual art consisting of four panels or figures, or dramatic works containing four temperamental characters, or musical works with four thematic movements. But four-part works of this kind are relatively rare. In music, which for quite unrelated reasons is the most amenable to four-part structures, this tradition has persisted into the modern period. For instance, Carl Nielsen (1865–1931) titled his Symphony no. 2 *The Four Temperaments* ('De fire temperamenter'), and gave each movement a tempo marker corresponding to one temperament: 'allegro collerico', 'allegro comodo e flemmatico', 'andante malinconico', and 'allegro sanguineo'. Likewise Paul Hindemith (1895–1963) composed a 'ballet for piano and strings' subtitled *The Four Temperaments*, with each temperament assigned to a separate variation. There is, however, a certain programmatic unwieldiness about works of this kind, which may explain their relative scarcity.

Where only one humour is represented, that humour is much more likely to be melancholia than the other three. This is chiefly because melancholia has a much wider field of application than the other three humours; the diversity of its uses is much greater; its cognitive and emotional content is more attractive. Music has a long-standing connection with melancholia, notably as a cure for it. Burton claimed to find examples of music curing melancholia in antiquity;[24] the most prominent example was David's driving out an evil spirit from Saul with his harp in 1 Samuel 16:23. Fashionable in Burton's day, melancholia became a popular theme in music. The most common melancholy form was song, but melancholy dance music was also popular. The 'Lachrimae' of John Dowland (1563–1626) was composed first as a pavan for the lute, and then adapted into the mournful song 'Flow My Tears'. From these beginnings melancholia developed into a familiar musical style. At least since Luigi Boccherini (1743–1805), *malinconico* or *con maliconia* has been used as a marker of tempo or mood, mainly for slow movements. Beethoven used it to describe the fourth movement of his String Quartet op. 18, no. 6, from which the quartet as a whole acquired the nickname 'La malinconia'. In the twentieth century, movements have been marked thus in works by Heitor Villa-Lobos (String Quartet no. 12), William Walton (Symphony no. 1), Camille Saint-Saëns (Introduction and Rondo Capriccioso op. 28 for Violin and Orchestra), and Owain Arwel Hughes (Symphony no. 1). There are whole works entitled melancholia by Francis Poulenc (*Mélancolie*, for solo piano), Emmanuel Chabrier ('Mélancolie', one of his *Pièces pittoresques* for solo piano), George Enescu (Andante malinconico for Violin and Piano), and Tiit Paulus (*Melanhoolne valss* ('Melancholy Waltz')). Another feature of this close connection between melancholia and music is that the descriptor *melancholy* has come to be used frequently in music appreciation and criticism, probably more so than in the other arts.

This brief and admittedly superficial account of melancholia in music could be repeated to similar effect for the visual arts. In literature the situation is significantly different. The influence of melancholia in literary culture has been much broader and much deeper than in music and art, for several reasons. First, because its medium is language, literature has more direct access to medical concepts than the visual arts and music do.

---

[24] Burton, *Anatomy*, vol. II, 114–16.

Second, during the Renaissance the term *melancholia* (or its cognates in other European languages) extended its use well beyond medicine and into ordinary discourse. The other temperament terms were also widely used in ordinary language, but they never achieved the same breadth of literary meaning as *melancholia*. The depressive realism hypothesis goes some way towards explaining why *melancholia* was so successful in literature. (The rest of this chapter provides examples, but only skims the surface.) Third, *melancholia* has a linguistic capacity that the sanguine, phlegmatic, and choleric humours have never had. *Melancholia* can act transitively. It is not just that a thing, indeed pretty much anything, can be described as having a melancholy feeling or mood. A melancholy thing can also impart its melancholy mood to the person experiencing it. When I refer to a melancholy scene, I might mean that the scene has a melancholy flavour. But I might also mean that it creates a melancholy mood in me. And often I would mean both. This sympathy between the melancholy flavour of an object and the melancholy mood of a subject is one reason why melancholy can apply so widely: to thoughts and ideas, to man-made and natural things, such as the built environment and landscape. The same does not happen with *sanguine, choleric,* and *phlegmatic*. It would be very odd to talk about a 'phlegmatic landscape', whereas a 'melancholy landscape' sounds perfectly natural, whether the landscape is in itself melancholy or whether it makes me feel melancholy (or both). So while the other three humours were also widely employed and they extended their usage well beyond medicine and into non-medical talk about character, *melancholia* was used much more frequently and widely. In eighteenth-century English texts, *melancholia* and its cognates occur twice as many times as all three other humours and their cognates put together.[25]

4   Melancholy philosophy

To explain the linguistic frequency of *melancholia*, we need to return to the notion of melancholy self-consciousness. If melancholia requires for its existence a culture of self-consciousness, and if it comes to have self-consciousness as one of its key contents, and if self-consciousness is a hallmark of Western culture, then it can be no surprise that melancholia has taken root in the West. Indeed, one way to look at cultural expressions of melancholia, as distinct from melancholia experienced as a disorder,

---

[25] The results of a search of *Eighteenth-Century Collections Online* (ECCO) for the following terms (with the number of hits in brackets): *melanchol** (66,457), *sanguin** (29,356), *choler** (12,745), and *phlegmat** (6,120).

is to see them as a peculiar intensification of self-consciousness. Melancholia is a way of being intensely self-conscious in art. Of course, intense self-consciousness need not always turn into melancholia. There are many rich forms of self-consciousness that lack the melancholy symptoms of sadness and anxiety. Melancholia is just one of the cultural forms that intense self-consciousness can take. One might think here of Lewis Wolpert's analogy between depression and cancer. Wolpert suggests that depression may be a malignant form of sadness.[26] Just as cancer cells are normal cells that divide and grow uncontrollably into malignant tumours, depression might be thought of as ordinary sadness that has mutated into an uncontrollable, virulent, and destructive form. Following Wolpert, we might call melancholia, at least in the kind of cultural expressions that concern us here, a malignant form of self-consciousness: a form of self-consciousness through which the self becomes harmful to itself.

How could melancholy self-consciousness come to have such malignant capacity? And why should a malignant form of self-consciousness be of special interest to writers and readers? In the first place, the cultural standing and the virulence of melancholia can be traced to trends in early modern philosophy. Melancholia was well suited to characterize (whether negatively or positively) pessimistic and sceptical styles of reasoning. For instance, melancholia could be a marker of virtuosity in the philosophical mystic or sceptic, as in Ficino's genial version of melancholia. Conversely, the pathological form of melancholia might be linked to excessive and undesirable scepticism or pessimism, in the same way as Luther and others accused some Protestant sectarians of melancholia. Either way, melancholia became entangled in philosophy and theology, and over time this made melancholia less susceptible to the traditional forms of moralizing critique. Traditional philosophical teaching stigmatized melancholics as sinful or nihilistic. If, however, melancholia was seen to be associated with a plausible philosophical stance, it might resist being written off so easily as mere psychopathology. Instead it might demand intellectual engagement. Second, melancholia has a well-documented tendency towards self-criticism, rehearsed in ceaseless circlings of self-critical rumination, which it shares with the practice of writing. Writing can be a miserably self-conscious activity. For some writers the melancholy mood has seemed a natural one in which to engage in self-criticism. A writer's melancholia might be connected with doubts about the writer's own creativity. And third, we have seen that melancholia has been intermittently fashionable. Rufus of Ephesus associated melancholia with the

---

[26] Lewis Wolpert, *Malignant Sadness: The Anatomy of Depression* (London: Faber and Faber, 1999).

admirable quality of high intelligence. *Problems* XXX/1, once rehabilitated by Ficino, gave melancholia a certain allure. But even before the birth of fashionable Renaissance melancholia, there was a dark glamour in being unhappy. As early as the fourteenth century, Petrarch could claim, 'I feed on my tears and grief with a sort of dark pleasure, so that it is only with great reluctance that I can tear myself away from them.'[27] It was the combination of melancholia's 'dark pleasure', its philosophical entanglements, and its capacity to feed creative self-criticism that made melancholy self-consciousness especially compelling for writers. This nexus of properties can be found in all periods of modern Western literature.

The history of melancholy philosophy, extending from the pseudo-Aristotelian *Problems* XXX/1 to Jean-Paul Sartre and beyond, can be viewed as a vindication of the depressive realism thesis, in theory if not in fact. Even if it did not in fact give philosophers any privileged access to the reality of human existence, melancholia was often thought to do so. Many thinkers and writers have believed in something a bit like depressive realism. From the Renaissance onwards, claims of this kind were made with increasing frequency and confidence. The author of *Problems* XXX/1 must at least have had an inkling of such a possibility when he decided to make philosophy prominent among the disciplines in which melancholics supposedly excelled. The author places philosophy first in the list of disciplines and gives us the names of three melancholy philosophers, Empedocles, Socrates, and Plato, though, admittedly, he does not tell us whether the melancholia was a fact about their disposition or about their philosophy. Given that the premise of the text is the link between melancholia and genius, one might infer that something in the content of the three philosophers' work must have appeared melancholy to the author of the *Problems*. However, he has nothing to say about the nature of any cognitive link between philosophy and melancholia. The classical tradition of melancholia had entertained the idea that philosophers were prone to melancholia because of the huge effort involved in philosophical cogitation. In the same way that physical exertion might wear out the body, mental exertion might exhaust the mind. Isḥāq ibn 'Imrān says that students of philosophy and science are especially prone to melancholia because of the stresses imposed by their object of study, in particular by 'brooding on the deeper meaning of things'.[28]

The idea of a cognitive link between melancholia and philosophy, as distinct from a physiological or habituated one, first emerges in Petrarch's

---

[27] Petrarch, *Secretum*, trans. J. G. Nichols (Richmond: Oneworld Classics, 2010), 60.
[28] Isḥāq ibn 'Imrān, *Maqāla fī'l-mālīhūliyā*, 14. The quotation is my translation of Garbers's German translation of ibn 'Imrān.

Secretum ('Secret Book', *c.* 1350), a fictive dialogue between Francisco (i.e. Petrarch) and St Augustine. Petrarch does not mention melancholia by name – the *Secretum* predates Ficino's rediscovery of the *Problems* by some 130 years. Petrarch was aware of the brief discussion of the *Problems* and its view of melancholy genius in Cicero's *Tusculan Disputations*, and Cicero's dialogue is one of Petrarch's main points of reference in the *Secretum*. The *Secretum* gives us a version of melancholia by another name and filtered through Cicero. Petrarch outlines the miserable condition from which Francisco suffers in terms very similar to melancholia: he has Augustine call it 'a spiritual bane, called by the moderns "acedia" and by the ancients *aegritudo* or sickness'.[29] The traditional Christian term *tristitia* (sadness) is also used, and this was the term with which medieval writers commonly translated *melancholia*. Because Francisco is a philosophically educated humanist, his malaise constitutes a challenge to Christian theology. At least that is how Petrarch's Augustine sees the matter. Certainly, the malaise has a Platonic flavour, for Francisco is constitutionally disdainful of all worldly things, and Augustine suggests that this disdain is one of the roots of the illness. In the *Secretum*, the malaise of *aegritudo–tristitia–melancholia* becomes the archetype of a certain style of philosophy.

One important source of Petrarch's philosophy was the mind–body dualism of the Platonic tradition, in particular the Neoplatonic philosopher Plotinus. According to Plotinus, man is composed of a divinely born soul that strives towards God but is shackled in melancholy union to an earthly body. Plotinus' view of man as radically decentred and distant from God was one ingredient of the new notion of melancholy genius, formulated by Ficino in the late fifteenth century.[30] Against this background of Renaissance Neoplatonist metaphysics, Ficino gives a markedly subjective account of melancholia. The typical melancholic is a person like himself, a scholar. Scholars are especially prone to melancholia, and among scholars philosophers are the most affected. Like Isḥāq ibn ʿImrān, Ficino believes that the effort involved in philosophizing is punishing and leads to melancholia. He further embeds the idea of the melancholy philosopher in a Neoplatonist version of the disease, according to which the cognitive content of philosophy causes melancholia. Philosophers are the living embodiment of mind–body dualism. Their minds are so fixed on incorporeal ideas that they become painfully separated from their bodies, so exacerbating the already melancholy human condition.[31]

---

[29] Petrarch, *Secretum*, 59.

[30] Marsilio Ficino, *The Book of Life*, trans. Charles Boer (Woodstock, CT: Spring, 1994), 86–91.

[31] Ficino, *The Book of Life*, 7.

Petrarch and Ficino were leading actors in one of the master plots of early modern philosophy: the Neoplatonist and humanist revolt against Aristotelian scholasticism. Both display the melancholy travails of this revolt, as well as its triumphs. Although the struggle to liberate mankind could be represented as heroically optimistic, some humanists were pessimistic, not least because they recognized that human understanding is prone to folly. Some Renaissance writers, notably Montaigne and Pascal, cultivated a self-image of the philosopher as a melancholy sceptic.[32] Burton went further and adopted the literary identity of 'Democritus Junior', disguising himself as a modern descendant of the Greek philosopher, who, according to one ancient tradition, had been mad.

For all their eminence, Petrarch, Ficino, Montaigne, and Pascal were in a small minority in finding philosophical meaning in melancholia. For most early modern philosophers, melancholia was incompatible with philosophical truth. While ancient writers like the author of the *Problems* and Rufus might have ascribed a certain intellectual brilliance to melancholics, the main philosophical schools of later antiquity, the Aristotelians and Stoics, viewed melancholia as a source of moral error, insofar as they acknowledged it at all. Most Renaissance thinkers followed the Aristotelian and Stoic line in viewing melancholia as morally obnoxious.[33] The seventeenth-century rationalists viewed the matter no differently. In his *Meditations* Descartes defended the rational procedure of scepticism by differentiating it from the errors produced by melancholy delusion.[34] Scepticism was philosophically serious and worth entertaining, if ultimately wrong; melancholia was a form of madness. Spinoza took a similarly dim view of melancholia. He presents his *Ethics* as, among other things, a cure for melancholia.[35]

The relationship between melancholia and philosophy changed decisively with the advent of sensibility and empirico-scepticism in the eighteenth century. Melancholia became associated with philosophical positions that were initially dangerous or unconventional but eventually became part of mainstream philosophy. David Hume, a master of philosophical brinkmanship, was also the melancholy philosopher *par*

---

[32] On Montaigne, see M. A. Screech, *Montaigne and Melancholy: The Wisdom of the Essays* (London: Duckworth, 1983).

[33] See the detailed documentation in Angus Gowland, 'The Ethics of Renaissance Melancholy', *Intellectual History Review* 18 (2008), 103–17.

[34] Réné Descartes, *The Philosophical Writings of Descartes*, trans. John Cottingham, Robert Stoothoff, and Dugald Murdoch, 3 vols. (Cambridge University Press, 1984–91), vol. II, 13.

[35] Willem Lemmens, 'Melancholy of the Philosopher: Hume and Spinoza on Emotions and Wisdom', *Journal of Scottish Philosophy* 3 (2005), 47–65.

excellence.[36] Hume had suffered from a series of bouts of melancholia in his youth. His medical history is recorded in a long letter to a physician, possibly Cheyne, from whom Hume sought advice on treatment for the disease.[37] But melancholia was not only a fact of Hume's biography: it was also a consciously, explicitly developed stage in his philosophical work. There is evidence of a melancholy scepticism throughout Hume's mature writings, and especially in his psychological demolition of religious belief in *The Natural History of Religion* (1757), which ends on a decidedly melancholy note.[38] Melancholia is also present in Hume's great statement of scepticism in *A Treatise of Human Nature* (1739–40). At the conclusion of Book I, Hume has established that personal identity is a mere fiction constructed by the imagination. Experience cannot rescue us from this melancholy truth, nor is the intellect a helpful guide, since, strictly applied, it leads only to complete scepticism 'either in philosophy or common life'.[39] From this bleak vantage point he reflects on 'those immense depths of philosophy, which lie before [him]' in his quest for an 'accurate anatomy of human nature':

Methinks I am like a man, who having struck on many shoals, and having narrowly escaped shipwreck in passing a small frith, has yet the temerity to put out to sea in the same leaky weather-beaten vessel, and even carries his ambition so far as to think of compassing the globe under these disadvantageous circumstances. My memory of past errors and perplexities, makes me diffident for the future. The wretched condition, weakness, and disorder of the faculties, I must employ in my enquiries, encrease my apprehensions. And the impossibility of amending or correcting these faculties, reduces me almost to despair, and makes me resolve to perish on the barren rock, on which I am at present, rather than venture myself upon that boundless ocean, which runs out into immensity. This sudden view of my danger strikes me with melancholy; and as it is usual for that passion, above all others, to indulge itself; I cannot forbear feeding my despair, with all those desponding reflections, which the present subject furnishes me with in such abundance.[40]

The symptoms of this melancholia are traditional: apprehension, fear, a sense of one's own inadequacy, rumination, and an indulgent languishing

---

[36] Livia Guimaraes, 'A Melancholy Skeptic', *Kriterion: Revista de Filosofia* 108 (2003), 180–90.

[37] David Hume, *The Letters of David Hume*, ed. J. Y. T. Greig, 2 vols. (Oxford University Press, 1932), vol. I, 12–18.

[38] David Hume, *Principal Writings on Religion Including 'Dialogues Concerning Natural Religion' and 'Natural History of Religion'*, ed. J. C. A. Gaskin (Oxford University Press, 1993), 184.

[39] David Hume, *A Treatise of Human Nature*, ed. L. A. Selby-Bigge, rev. P. H. Nidditch (Oxford University Press, 1978), 267–8.

[40] *Ibid.*, 263–4.

in precisely those emotions that melancholia generates. Worse is to follow. The philosopher's sceptical rumination is a solitary activity and leads to alienation from society. The sceptical stance is unacceptable to most people, and Hume returns the compliment by finding society disgustingly shallow. Melancholia has set in, accompanied by its usual symptoms of delusions, hesitation, and dread. All that can be done is to treat the melancholia with one of the traditional cures, amusement and diversion:

> Most fortunately it happens, that since reason is incapable of dispelling these clouds, nature herself suffices to that purpose, and cures me of this philosophical melancholy and delirium, either by relaxing this bent of mind, or by some avocation, and lively impression of my senses, which obliterate all these chimeras. I dine, I play a game of back-gammon, I converse, and am merry with my friends; and when after three or four hours' amusement, I would return to these speculations, they appear so cold, and strained, and ridiculous, that I cannot find in my heart to enter into them any farther.[41]

Though the melancholy scepticism might now strike Hume as absurd, it has not gone away. Far from conquering the melancholy truths, Hume has only found temporary relief from them.

From the middle of the eighteenth century, melancholia began to insinuate itself into the heart of the Enlightenment project. There were always (at least) two impulses in the philosophy of the Enlightenment. One was the impulse to eradicate illusions, whether the illusions of revealed religion or of an overly ambitious rationalism. By destroying illusions, philosophers hoped to clear the decks and rebuild truth on a secure, anthropocentric foundation. By replacing theological and metaphysical illusion with anthropological truth, humans could take charge of their destiny. This was the second pillar of the Enlightenment, the struggle to become autonomous, which was often expressed in terms of the Delphic injunction to 'know thyself'. But as Hume's example shows, demolished illusions might create a space that would fill not with confident personal autonomy, but with a diffuse sense of melancholy anxiety.[42] This was not a purely passive process. It was bound up with human freedom, the freedom to remove illusions, to question authority and tradition. For freedom could bring with it a sense of 'dizziness', as Kierkegaard would later observe.[43] The Enlightenment worked to

---

[41] *Ibid.*, 269.
[42] Christian Begemann, *Furcht und Angst im Prozeß der Aufklärung: zu Literatur und Bewußtseinsgeschichte des 18. Jahrhunderts* (Frankfurt/Main: Athenäum, 1987).
[43] 'anxiety is the dizziness of freedom', Søren Kierkegaard, *The Concept of Anxiety*, trans. Reidar Thomte (Princeton University Press, 1980), 61.

establish the limits of our possible knowledge, and in the process discovered the melancholy truth that our limits are in some sense imperfections. Diderot put it crisply in his article 'Mélancolie' in the *Encyclopédie*: 'MELANCHOLY: this is the habitual feeling of our own imperfection'.[44] The melancholy sense of human imperfection, accompanied by sudden flashes of fear or background rumblings of anxiety, would become ingrained in modern European thought, and would be elaborated in painful detail by Schopenhauer, Nietzsche, William James, Walter Benjamin, and Jean-Paul Sartre, to name only a few.

5   Melancholia and modern poetics

The same melancholy sense of human imperfection became even more deeply ingrained in modern literature. To some extent literary melancholia piggybacked on philosophy, but it was able to go further and faster down the road to melancholia because it was bound to a lesser extent than philosophy by the imperatives of truth and usefulness. In early modern theatre, philosophical rumination became a key indicator of the melancholy temperament. The content of the rumination often had noble philosophical ancestry. It was circumstances that taught Hamlet to think sceptically about the conventional pieties of statecraft and religion, and more generally about the inconstancy of human character. But the expression of his scepticism depended very much on the philosophical culture of humanism, such as the sceptical humanism of Montaigne, whom Shakespeare may have read in the translation by his friend John Florio. Hamlet's melancholy ruminations on the uncertainties of our existence were reprised in later dramatic recreations of the Danish prince. Schiller's hesitant and melancholy Wallenstein ruminates grandly but emptily. As the net fabricated out of his own conspiracies closes over him, Wallenstein ponders whether we can ever really determine our actions; like Hamlet, he weighs existence against suicide ('What? I, no longer as I might choose?').[45] Goethe's Faust, a melancholy scholar in the manner of Ficino, also reprises Hamlet's meditations. Faust broods on how we are locked into our fate by crude materiality: our idealistic aspirations get clogged with cruft; the flight of the imagination is hobbled by anxiety. Braver and more certain of his own convictions than Hamlet, Faust

---

[44] 'MÉLANCOLIE: *C'est le sentiment habituel de notre imperfection*', in Denis Diderot and Jean le Rond d'Alembert (eds.), *Encyclopédie, ou Dictionnaire raisonné des sciences, des arts et des métiers* (Paris: Briasson *et al.*, 1751–72), vol. XXI, 415.

[45] Friedrich Schiller, *Wallenstein's Death*, Act I, scene iv, in Schiller, *The Robbers and Wallenstein*, 328.

decides on suicide and is only saved by the fortuitous singing of a nearby choir on Easter morning.

The allure of melancholy philosophizing is realized nowhere with greater power than in Goethe's *Werther*. Here the link to philosophical melancholia is strikingly obvious both within the text and in the circumstances of its genesis. A few months before the novel's publication, Goethe wrote to a friend, describing Werther as 'a young person, who is gifted with deep, pure sensibility and real penetration... [He] gets lost in fantastical dreams, undermines himself with speculation, until finally, on top of it all he is shattered by unhappy passion, in particular an unfulfillable love, and shoots himself in the head.'[46] Partly autobiographical, the character of Werther was also based on a young would-be philosopher Goethe had known since his student days, Karl Wilhelm Jerusalem. The style of philosophy Jerusalem practised was, unusually for Germany at the time, strongly influenced by Hume. Jerusalem wrote an essay in defence of suicide similar to Hume's posthumously published 'On Suicide', which had been circulating in clandestine copies since 1770. Taking his lead from Jerusalem's philosophical leanings, Goethe imagines Werther as a thoroughgoing Humean sceptic and melancholic. He insists on the limits of our knowledge, rejects universals, argues for the sensuous origin of all ideas, and claims that suicide is the result of illness, not moral defect. All of this is presented, moreover, in a manner designed to appeal to the contemporary taste for sensibility. Werther writes in an unbuttoned style marked by regional dialect and archaisms; he seems to speak spontaneously and from the heart; he delivers a fashionable Rousseauian critique of civilization. His melancholy philosophy is wrapped in a fatally glamorous package.

A distinction emerged in the eighteenth century between 'black' melancholia and 'white' melancholia. The former, genuinely medical and pathological, was accompanied by profound terrors.[47] The latter was a gentler, more poetic, and presumably affected form. The distinction is somewhat misleading, however, inasmuch as it implies that only white melancholia was pleasurable. Black melancholia could also be pleasurable, as the self-portrayals of Petrarch, Hume, and Goethe's Werther demonstrate. Indeed, it could be argued that the pain of melancholia was precisely what brought pleasure. To put it another way, the relation between melancholia, pain and pleasure, and performance is a complex one. Instead of the black/white model, it may be more helpful to distinguish between two forms of melancholy pleasure, both of which could be

[46] Goethe to G. F. A. Schönborn, June 1774, in Johann Wolfgang Goethe, *Werke*, ed. Erich Schmidt *et al.*, 146 vols. (Weimar: Böhlau, 1887–1919), vol. IV, 2, 171.
[47] Sickels, *The Gloomy Egoist*, 66–7.

performed, poeticized, and potentially trivialized. One form is the melancholy jollity we find in sixteenth- and seventeenth-century literature. The other is Petrarch's 'dark pleasure' or Hume's 'passion' that 'indulge[s] itself', in other words an indulgent fascination with genuine pain. The melancholy jollity of the Elizabethan and Jacobean era was closely associated with mirth. The melancholic would experience sudden shifts between sadness and jollity. Many authorities, Burton included, insisted that melancholics were capable of exceptional wit. It is no accident that the word 'humour' developed an ambiguous meaning at this time, referring both to a person's temperament and to wit itself. So Shakespeare's melancholy Jaques in *As You Like It* talks punningly of his 'most humorous sadness' (Act IV, scene i).[48] On one definition, wit was marked by sudden shifts into and out of temperament. One measure of wit was the rapidity with which a character changed mood. Melancholy poems are often marked by this duality. In the dialogic poem that prefaces Burton's *Anatomy*, the stanzas alternate between two claims about the relation between melancholia, pain, and pleasure: melancholia is both the most pleasurable ('All my joyes to this are folly, / Naught so sweet as melancholy') and painful condition ('All my griefes to this are jolly, / Naught so fierce as melancholy').[49] Milton's vision of melancholia in 'Il Penseroso' is paired with a vision of mirth in 'L'Allegro'.

These highly stylized seventeenth-century versions of the melancholy pain–pleasure dichotomy, while on the surface quite different, were in fact related to Petrarch's 'dark pleasure'. This became clearer in the eighteenth century with the emergence of the idea that pain was closely related to pleasure. The dominant psychological model of the eighteenth century was based on stimulus, whether pleasurable or painful. As both pain and pleasure were forms of stimulus, pain could be understood as the flipside of pleasure. Indeed, pain could be thought to contain some pleasure. As a literary trope, this became especially popular after the publication of MacPherson's 'Ossian' poems. It was MacPherson who coined the phrase 'joy of grief' – it was 'one of Ossian's remarkable expressions, several times repeated', as MacPherson's friend and supporter Hugh Blair noted in his *Critical Dissertation on the Poems of Ossian* (1763). In order to lend the phrase authority, Blair traced it back to Homer, though, like the Ossian phenomenon itself, the phrase was transparently a product of the age of sensibility. Feeling, any feeling, was primary, even if the feeling was grief.[50]

---

[48] Shakespeare, *As You Like It*, 95.
[49] Burton, *Anatomy*, 'The Authors Abstract of Melancholy', vol. I, lxix–lxxi.
[50] Hugh Blair, *Critical Dissertation on the Poems of Ossian* (London: Becket and De Hondt, 1763), 150.

A corollary of this close relation of joy to grief is that the dichotomy of affect can be cut in a new way. Instead of setting grief in opposition to joy, one could set grief and joy on one side of the dichotomy and an absence of any feeling on the other. This is what some eighteenth-century advocates of sensibility did. Joy is best, grief second best, and an absence of feeling worst. In other words, feeling grief is preferable to feeling nothing. From this it follows that feelings of melancholy affect could be a source of pleasure in an otherwise 'weary, stale, flat, and unprofitable ... world'. This is one source of the much derided propensity of literary figures in the age of sensibility to weep apparently at the slightest provocation. (Editing MacKenzie's *The Man of Feeling* in 1886, Henry Morley added an 'Index of Tears' containing a full forty-seven references, even though he forbore to include 'Chokings, etc.')[51] Tears have value for the melancholic because they indicate an ability to feel, and that is surely preferable to no feeling at all. In this spirit Goethe's Werther begs for tears as a form of release from his emotional numbness:

And now that heart is dead and no longer gives me joy, my eyes are dry, and my senses are not refreshed by heartfelt tears any more but furrow my brow with fearful worries. I suffer a great deal because I have lost the sole pleasure in my life, that sacred and inspiring power to create new worlds about me; – it is gone! When I gaze from my window at the distant hills and see the morning sun breaking through the mist above them and shining through the tranquil meadows, and the river gently meandering amongst the leafless willows – Oh! all the glories of Nature are frozen to my eye, like a varnished painting, and all the delights are powerless to extract one drop of joy from my heart to refresh my mind, and there I stand, in the sight of God, like a dried-up spring, like a broken pitcher. I have often prostrated myself on the ground and prayed to God for tears, like a farmer praying for rain when the heaven over his head is brass and the earth is parched.[52]

The ability to weep is a sign of the ability to feel and is therefore closely related to aesthetic sensibility and to our capacity to be moved by the beauties of nature and art. In this sense too, joy is the partner of grief.

From the joy of grief it is a small step to the grief of joy and to the melancholy awareness that any pleasure contains its own grief. In Keats's 'Ode on Melancholy', melancholia becomes fully aestheticized. Melancholia is the grief residing within the evanescent experience of pleasure. If you want to find true melancholy, Keats seems to say, seek the fleetingness of beauty:

[51] Markman Ellis, *The Politics of Sensibility: Race, Gender and Commerce in the Sentimental Novel* (Cambridge University Press, 1996), 19.
[52] Goethe, *Werther*, 98.

Ay, in the very temple of Delight
  Veil'd Melancholy has her sovran shrine,
    Though seen of none save him whose strenuous tongue
Can burst Joy's grape against his palate fine;
    His soul shall taste the sadness of her might,
    And be among her cloudy trophies hung.[53]

The onset of melancholia in Keats's poem is marked by a sudden tearful fall: 'when the melancholy fit shall fall / Sudden from heaven like a weeping cloud'. Likewise the melancholy aesthete enjoys an instantaneous pleasure in bursting the grape. This suddenness has both emotional and cognitive dimensions. In emotional terms, the onset of melancholia is marked by a sudden drop into melancholy affect. In cognitive terms, there is a sudden realization of the melancholy truth about the world.

The fall into melancholy affect is frequently found in the form of dramatic pathos. In drama melancholia can mark a final and tragic change of fortunes, an irreversible shift into the tragic mode. This is a characteristic feature in the plays of Friedrich Schiller, several of which end by pitching us into an atmosphere of melancholia, as hard, bitter fate makes the characters aware of the hopelessness or futility of their ideals. For instance, in his second play, *The Conspiracy of Fiesco in Genoa*, the hero's young wife Leonore charges into the chaotic streets of revolutionary Genoa, having given up hope of defeating 'the black breath of grief', as she describes her own melancholia.[54] As Don Cesar puts it in *The Bride of Messina*, the self-destructive urge arises when we realize that death is the only way 'to eradicate the flaws of impure / Humanity'.[55] In *Wallenstein's Death*, Wallenstein's daughter, Thekla, laments the end of her hopes of marriage to the brave and idealistic Max Piccolomini:

It seemed the bliss of heaven should be my part,
My first awakened glance fell on your heart.
(*She falls silent, pensive, then starts up with an expression of horror.*)
Then cold and grim must destiny appear,
Must seize the tender shape of him so dear
And cast him under his horses' galloping hooves.
All beauty on this earth fate thus reproves![56]

---

[53] John Keats, *Poetical Works*, ed. H. W. Garrod (Oxford University Press, 1989), 220.

[54] Friedrich Schiller, *Die Verschwörung des Fiesco zu Genua*, Act IV, scene xiv, in Schiller, *Werke*. Nationalausgabe, ed. Julius Petersen *et al.* (Stuttgart: Böhlau, 1943 ff.), vol. IV, 102.

[55] Schiller, *Die Braut von Messina*, lines 2734–5, in Schiller, *Werke*. Nationalausgabe, vol. X, 121.

[56] Schiller, *Wallenstein*, 443 (lines 3175–80).

As in Keats's ode, beauty reminds us of impermanence. Often the head-long pitch into melancholy affect is accompanied by a cognitive shock, a pathos of realization, akin to the sublime, only with melancholia replacing the disorientating or uplifting feelings that usually accompany the sublime. Whereas the sublime confronts us with a universe that exceeds our capacity to comprehend it, the melancholy sublime contains a sudden realization that the world is not far greater than we can comprehend but far sadder or more terrifying than we can cope with. We fall suddenly from an ordinary and relatively comfortable view of the world into an appreciation of its melancholy terror. Goethe's Werther provides a striking instance of this when he describes how his view of nature as a creative, pantheistic paradise suddenly switched into a terrifying morbid hell. The sudden shift is expressed in terms of a curtain being drawn to reveal the grisly scene beyond: 'It is as if a curtain had been drawn from before my soul, and this scene of infinite life had been transformed before my eyes into the abyss of the grave, forever open wide.'[57] In Werther's melancholy sublime, nature is deadly and destructive, constantly devouring what it produces. With less affect but no less impact, Byron defines melancholia as the effect of suddenly focusing in on reality as if with a telescope, in his 1816 poem 'The Dream':

> [T]he wise
> Have a far deeper madness – and the glance
> Of melancholy is a fearful gift;
> What is it but the telescope of truth?
> Which strips the distance of its fantasies,
> And brings life near in utter nakedness,
> Making the cold reality too real![58]

Werther's curtain and Byron's telescope are metaphors for essentially one and the same process. A comfortable and habituated illusion suddenly gives way to a terrifying reality. Or it may be that one reality makes way for another. In Victor Hugo's poem 'Saturn', the speaker claims that his own melancholy vision of the world has been seen by prophets and mystics since the days of the patriarchs. These visionaries are haunted by the knowledge of a world that is suddenly and fitfully revealed through a fissure torn open in reality. What is revealed is an 'obscure world of pale visions'.[59] Hugo's vision suggests a different sort of melancholy reality

[57] Goethe, *Werther*, 66.
[58] George Gordon, Lord Byron, *Works. Poetry*, vol. VI, ed. Ernest Hartley Coleridge (London: Murray, 1905), 40.
[59] 'le monde obscur des pâles visions', Victor Hugo, 'Saturne', in Hugo, *Œuvres Poétiques*, ed. Pierre Albouy, 3 vols. (Paris: Gallimard, 1964–74), vol. II, 580.

from the horror that shocked Werther, more Romantic ennui than pre-Romantic Gothic terror. It shares some of the character of Keats's 'cloudy trophies': insubstantial, uncertain, featureless. The shock of the perceptual shift gives way to a sad knowledge that there is actually not much to see, or at least not much to enjoy.

Since romanticism, and arguably even before, the idea of a privileged insight into reality has been a core doctrine in the creed of the poet. But privileged insight comes at a cost. To see things differently is to risk alienation from common modes of thought and being. The poet's insight may be bought at the cost of his isolation. The upside is that the poet's insight may offer some consolation. The depressive realism hypothesis contains a similar thought. If depressed cognition generates a more accurate picture of reality, those who suffer from depression can at least console themselves with the thought that they see the world more clearly than those who are healthy. Keats's ode offers the poetic version of this idea. 'Delight' is only accessible to the aesthete 'whose strenuous tongue / Can burst Joy's grape against his palate fine', but who is condemned to melancholia for his pains. The idea that poetic insight was bought at a cost reached its peak in German modernism, as J. P. Stern has shown. The fate of the artist is to become aware of 'a salvation or validation of man which is to be attained at the highest price that man can conceive of':

While at times the price exacted is beyond – tantalizingly just beyond – what a man can pay with his entire being and existence. It is a salvation whose very validity is relative to its being supremely difficult of attainment, or even (in its most radical formulation) to its unattainableness. And, conversely, anything that is not attained at such exorbitant cost cannot be the real thing at all: It is either rejected outright, or it is presented in a radically different light.[60]

For poets from romanticism onwards, consolation for melancholia came in the form of aesthetic experience itself. The price was, in one way or another, worth paying. In his 'Ballad of the Outer Life' ('Ballade des äußeren Lebens') Hugo von Hofmannsthal (1874–1929) details the melancholy emptiness of the everyday:

> And the wind blows, and we hear the sound
> Of words and over and over repeat their sense
> And feel desire both weary and profound.[61]

---

[60] J. P. Stern, 'The Dear Purchase', *German Quarterly* 41 (1968), 317–37 (at p. 321); for a full exposition, see Stern, *The Dear Purchase: A Theme in German Modernism* (Cambridge University Press, 1995).

[61] Hugo von Hofmannsthal, 'Ballad of the Outer Life', in *The Whole Difference: Selected Writings of Hugo von Hofmannsthal*, ed. J. D. McClatchy (Princeton University Press, 2008), 29. I have adapted the translation.

Life's random and ceaseless comings and goings seem empty of purpose. The only consolation is the aesthetic experience of melancholia itself in the utterance of the word 'evening', one of melancholia's traditional icons:

> What good is all of this to us, this game?
> However great we grow, we are lonely still
> And wander the world without an aim.
>
> To learn merely this, we leave our homes?
> And he says everything who just says 'evening',
> A word from which the richest sadness spills
>
> Like heavy honey from the hollow combs.

Melancholy alienation can be redeemed through aesthetic experience. A less romantic and less confident idea of the redemptive or consolatory power of poetry occurs in T. S. Eliot's 'melancholy tone-poem' *The Waste Land*.[62] Eliot's patchwork poem remorselessly documents the spiritual and emotional brokenness of modern life, from which there seems to be no escape. For the poet overcome by this melancholy sense of fragmentation, the most plausible response is to create a poem that is itself composed of fragments. *The Waste Land* mixes fragments of experience with fragments of the literary tradition. The poem ends with a characteristic concatenation of fragments from diverse sources. Inserted within these is a vision of the poet constructing his own consolatory fragmentary work:

> I sat upon the shore
> Fishing, with the arid plain behind me
> Shall I at least set my lands in order?
>
> London Bridge is falling down falling down falling down
>
> *Poi s'ascose nel foco che gli affina*
> *Quando fiam uti chelidon* – O swallow swallow
> *Le Prince d'Aquitaine à la tour abolie*
> These fragments I have shored against my ruins
> Why then Ile fit you. Hieronymo's mad againe.
> Datta. Dayadhvam. Damyata.
>
> *Shantih shantih shantih.* (lines 423–33)[63]

---

[62] Eliot's friend Conrad Aiken termed *The Waste Land* a 'powerful, melancholy tone-poem' in his review of 1923. Aiken later reported that Eliot had angrily rejected the label 'melancholy', though he did accept that the title of Aiken's review, 'An Anatomy of Melancholy', was apt given the amount of quotation in *The Waste Land* and Burton's *Anatomy*. The review and the story of Eliot's reaction can be found in Conrad Aiken, 'An Anatomy of Melancholy', *Sewanee Review* 74 (1966), 188–96 (at pp. 189–90).

[63] T. S. Eliot, *Collected Poems 1909–1935* (London: Faber & Faber, 1936), 77.

6   Melancholy deserts

With his back to the 'arid plain', Eliot's poet sits in a properly melancholy location. In this final section, I look briefly at the topos of the desert, one of the many literary topoi that have been associated with melancholia. The 'waste land' depicted in Eliot's poem is a desert in two senses: in the modern geographical sense of being a land without water or vegetation ('the arid plain'), and in the older sense of being a deserted and abandoned land ('The wind / Crosses the brown land, unheard. The nymphs are departed', lines 174–5). The former sense symbolizes the emotional aridity of the modern individual, which the poem has played out above all in part III, 'The Fire Sermon'. A brief sexual liaison is observed by the ancient Tiresias, 'old man with wrinkled dugs', against the background of a desolate London. The latter sense of desolation and desertedness is conveyed throughout by the poem's textural structure, in which exotic fragments of older poetic traditions are set within the flatter idioms of modernity.

From the beginnings of the Western tradition the desert was seen as the natural site of melancholia. In the medical literature deserted places were linked with the melancholic's love of solitude. In a text traditionally attributed to Galen, the Byzantine physician Aëtius of Amida says that 'many [melancholics] wish to frequent dark places and ruins and solitude'.[64] Du Laurens writes that melancholics are found 'straying and wandring in solitarie places'.[65] In some cases the solitude of the desert brings on melancholia. According to Burton, 'desart places cause melancholy in an instant'.[66] Indeed, deserts illustrate the double sense of melancholia that we saw in section 3 above: they are melancholy in themselves, and they have the power to cause melancholy in those who experience them. From causing melancholia, deserts came to symbolize it, or, more accurately, they came to represent melancholy visions of existence. The desert represented the way the melancholic saw the world, literally 'weary, stale, flat, and unprofitable'. As well as reminding us of the solitude of man, they symbolize the transience of all worldly things. All lands have a tendency to revert to desert if not properly tended, and so they suffer the transience and vanity to which all human effort is prone.

The idea of barrenness has been especially powerful in the Judaeo-Christian tradition, where the desert is a sign of God's departure from a

---

[64] [Aëtius], *De Melancholia*, in Galen, *Opera Omnia*, ed. C. G. Kühn, 20 vols. (Leipzig: Knobloch, 1821–33), vol. XIX, 702.

[65] Du Laurens, *Discourse*, 80.   [66] Burton, *Anatomy*, vol. I, p. 237.

world made unproductive by man's sin. God's creation was naturally fruitful, but the sin of Adam and Eve ended this fruitfulness ('cursed [is] the ground for thy sake', Genesis 3:17). The Humans were cast out of Eden into a world that required the hard labour of cultivation, without which the land would revert to desert ('in sorrow shalt thou eat [of] it all the days of thy life. Thorns also and thistles shall it bring forth to thee', Genesis 3:17–18). The desert was therefore a reminder of God's abandonment of man. In the Christian tradition the desert also became a place of withdrawal, renunciation, and spiritual struggle. Christ retired to the desert and fought off the temptations of Satan. Building on these Graeco-Roman and Judaeo-Christian traditions, later writers would derive from the desert their own melancholy insights into moments of decline or crisis.

Early writers on melancholia were able to cite even more ancient cases of melancholics seeking out desert solitude. The pseudo-Aristotelian *Problems* XXX/1 begins by quoting lines from the *Iliad*, Book VI, which describe the outcast hero Bellerophontes wandering across the empty plains of Aleion:

> But after Bellerophontes was hated by all the immortals,
> He wandered alone about the plain of Aleïon,
> Eating his heart out, skulking aside from the trodden track of
>   humanity.[67]

Although melancholia is not mentioned in this passage or indeed anywhere in the Homeric epics, the wanderings of Bellerophontes became an icon of the disease, thanks to the author of the *Problems* XXX/1. Other mythical or legendary figures might have served the purpose just as well. Had it been a part of their tradition, Graeco-Roman and later Western authors could have cited the case of Gilgamesh that we discussed in Chapter 1. In mourning for the death of his friend Enkidu, Gilgamesh abandons his people and wanders in the wilderness. There he meets several supernatural figures who comment on his appearance and behaviour, among them Ur-shanabi, ferryman of the river of the dead:

> Ur-shanabi spoke to him, to Gilgamesh,
> 'Why are your cheeks wasted, your face dejected,
> Your heart so wretched, your appearance worn out,
> And grief in your innermost being?
> Your face is like that of a long-distance traveller.
> Your face is weathered by cold and heat . . .
> Clad only in a lion-skin, you roam open country.'[68]

---

[67] Homer, *Iliad*, 6, 200–3.   [68] *Gilgamesh*, 103.

The theme of the dejected prince wandering in the desert is also found in the Judaeo-Christian tradition. As we saw in Chapter 4, the New England Puritans found a special meaning in Psalm 107's description of the wanderings of the children of Israel. The text seemed to give voice to their own experience of religious melancholia in the New World. In the same Psalm we find the theme of the dejected prince wandering in the desert: 'Again, they are minished and brought low through oppression, affliction,. and sorrow. He poureth contempt upon princes, and causeth them to wander in the wilderness, where there is no way' (Psalms 107: 39–40). The trope of pathlessness brings the idea of leadership into sharp focus. The dejected or melancholy prince is, for a while at least, a failure as a leader. Because he has abandoned himself to solitude, the prince is not capable of giving proper leadership to his people. The desert is the appropriate place for his solitude as it lacks any human imprint or cultivation. The lack of paths in the desert signifies aimlessness, a loss of direction, and poor leadership. It is exactly where a good leader should not be.

A particularly expressive version of the motif of the prince in the pathless waste occurs in J. R. R. Tolkien's *The Lord of the Rings*. The 'crownless' king Aragorn is heir to the throne of Gondor, though he is not recognized as king, and Gondor has had no king for centuries. Instead Aragorn has spent his life ranging the northern wastelands of Middle-earth far from Gondor, a leader bereft of kingship. Indeed, Aragorn seems reluctant to take up his responsibilities. One of the plots of *The Lord of the Rings* concerns Aragorn's gradual discovery of his true vocation to lead the free peoples of Middle-earth. The first sign of his doing so is when he joins up with the Hobbits carrying Sauron's ring to temporary safety in Rivendell, and guides them through the trackless wilderness. In fairness to Aragorn, his reluctance to be king is not only a personal failing. It is one among many symptoms of a sadness that haunts the whole of Middle-earth. As the party hides from Sauron's Black Riders below the ruins of the watchtower of Amon Sûl, Aragorn sings the tale of Lúthien Tinúviel to the hobbits. 'It is a fair tale', he remarks, 'though it is sad, as are all the tales of Middle-earth.'[69] Aragorn cannot protect the Hobbits from the Black Riders' assault on Amon Sûl. Frodo is stabbed with a poisoned blade. A shard of the blade breaks off in his shoulder and begins to work its way towards his heart, threatening to subject him to Sauron. At this point, as the party trudges slowly through the wilderness carrying the wounded Frodo towards Rivendell, Aragorn reaches his lowest ebb:

[69] J. R. R. Tolkien, *The Lord of the Rings* (London: HarperCollins, 1995), 187.

They made their way slowly and cautiously round the south-western slopes of the hill, and came in a little while to the edge of the Road. There was no sign of the Riders. But even as they were hurrying across they heard far away two cries: a cold voice calling and a cold voice answering. Trembling they sprang forward, and made for the thickets that lay ahead. The land before them sloped away southwards, but it was wild and pathless; bushes and stunted trees grew in dense patches with wide barren spaces in between. The grass was scanty, coarse, and grey; and the leaves in the thickets were faded and falling. It was a cheerless land, and their journey was slow and gloomy. They spoke little as they trudged along. Frodo's heart was grieved as he watched them walking beside him with their heads down, and their backs bowed under their burdens. Even Strider [i.e. Aragorn] seemed tired and heavy-hearted.[70]

The passage is symptomatic of the melancholy condition of Middle-earth. The environment of Middle-earth has been poisoned by Sauron of Mordor and the treacherous wizard Saruman of Isengard. Mordor is now 'ruinous and dead, a desert burned and choked'.[71] Isengard's trees have been chopped down and its land adulterated by the 'filth' of Saruman.[72] Middle-earth has been all but abandoned by the Elves, its most beautiful creatures. The Ents, the oldest of its creatures, are no longer capable of reproducing. Men are losing their nobility and longevity. Settlements that once thrived are now derelict. When Gandalf is asked what will survive – 'may it not so end that much that was fair and wonderful shall pass forever out of Middle-earth?'– he acknowledges that 'the evil of Sauron cannot be wholly cured, nor made as if it had not been'.[73] And even though the Hobbits finally succeed in destroying Sauron's ring and Aragorn returns as king to Gondor, Gandalf's melancholy answer proves true. Frodo cannot be cured of his knife wound and leaves Middle-earth with the last of the Elves to live with his pain in the Undying Lands.

A stock topos of melancholy writing, the trackless waste has been adapted to a variety of historical circumstances and uses. Tolkien wrote after the experience of mechanized trench warfare in World War I. In the wake of the French Terror, 150 years before Tolkien's novel, the trackless waste could symbolize the destruction of the radical hopes briefly encouraged by the French Revolution. In his 1796 epic *Joan of Arc*, Robert Southey describes how the French defending Orléans scorched the surrounding territory:

> [W]ithout the walls the desolate plain
> Stretch'd wide, a rough and melancholy waste.
> With uptorn pavements and foundations deep
> Of many a ruined dwelling – horrid scene![74]

[70] *Ibid.*, 194.   [71] *Ibid.*, 902.   [72] *Ibid.*, 555.   [73] *Ibid.*, 537.
[74] Robert Southey, *The Poetical Works of Robert Southey, Collected by Himself*, 10 vols. (Longman: London, 1837), vol. I, 77.

Twenty years later, Wordsworth's poem 'Composed in Recollection of the Expedition of the French into Russia, *February 1816*' contains a lament for the French legions retreating from Moscow:

> Distracted, spiritless, benumbed, and blind,
> Whole legions sink – and, in one instant, find
> Burial and death: look for them – and descry,
> When morn returns, beneath the clear blue sky,
> A soundless waste, a trackless vacancy!

The melancholy pathless wasteland is the outcome of man's self-destructive potential.

Also a token of man's capacity for self-destruction, albeit on an individual scale, the trackless waste appears as a topos of love melancholia. Perhaps the first use of the motif in this context is Petrarch's sonnet 'Solo e pensoso i più deserti campi'. Petrarch presents himself trying to escape love, but it follows him everywhere, even into the deserted wilderness: 'Alone and filled with care, I go / Measuring the most deserted fields with steps delaying and slow.'[75] In a more self-destructive vein, Goethe's poem 'Winter Journey in the Harz' ('Harzreise im Winter', 1777) features a misanthropic victim of love melancholia. His destructive passion has driven him into the wilderness where he 'consumes unseen / His own value's core'. Just as the poet catches sight of him, perhaps hoping to bring consolation, the figure disappears into the undergrowth:

> See, his path is lost in the scrub,
> Hard on his footsteps
> The bushes are closing,
> The grass springs back again,
> The wasteland devours him.[76]

---

[75] *Petrarch's Lyric Poems*, trans. Robert M. Durling (Cambridge, MA: Harvard University Press, 1976), 94.

[76] Goethe, 'Harzreise im Winter', in *Selected Poems*, trans. John Whaley (London: J. M. Dent, 1998), 41.

Conclusion

The melancholic disappears into the wasteland. Melancholics often do disappear, retreating into isolation or taking their own lives. But to imagine that melancholia itself could disappear, as is surely the hope of Goethe's poem 'Winter Journey in the Harz', is particularly wishful. (In fairness, sometimes Goethe tried to write melancholia into oblivion, but more often he accommodated it.) In any case, melancholia will not go away. It is not only a disorder suffered discretely by individuals the length and breadth (more or less) of the Western tradition. Melancholia is also an inalienable feature of Western culture. It has become so because Western culture has, at least for large parts of its history since fifth-century BC Greece, accorded a high status to self-consciousness. We can only explain the reality and durability of melancholia by looking into the heart of our self-conscious culture. Stanley Jackson concludes his history of melancholia with these words: 'with such distress, we are at the very heart of being human'.[1] I would say rather: with the distress of melancholia we are at the very heart of being human in the West.

What are the advantages of the self-consciousness model of melancholia set out in these pages? And what difficulties does it create? Jackson has argued that the core psychological symptoms of melancholia have an underlying reality, and that this explains their durability. Questions remain concerning the nature of this reality. Does melancholia deserve to count as a disease in a formal nosological sense, or is it better imagined as a regularly co-occurring cluster of symptoms? Important as they are, these questions have little bearing on the self-consciousness model. What matters for our purposes is that the symptoms have been observed and experienced regularly right across the historical span of Western culture from the fifth century BC to the present day. Melancholia has been with us for 2,500 years.

Since melancholia first appeared as a nosological category in the Hippocratic writings 2,500 years ago, it has been usual to lump the symptoms together as a single entity. Why should the symptoms be visible

---

[1] Jackson, *Melancholia*, 404.

to us in this particular way? Why have we continued to lump them together? The lumping of melancholia depends on a particular way of doing science. It depends on our being interested in putting things into classes, rather than treating each individual instance as *sui generis*. Since the scientific revolution in sixth-century BC Greek Ionia, we have tended to class natural phenomena together into kinds, and we have sought naturalistic causal explanations for their belonging together. In this sense melancholia is a product of a particular way of doing science that emerged in sixth-century BC Greece. Although philosophers continue to debate the possibility and nature of natural kinds, no better way of doing science has successfully challenged the Ionian scientific method.

Kinds of things need labels, and the whys and wherefores of labelling are complex. The most important factors are descriptive aptness, metaphorical richness, and the authority of tradition. The origins of the word *melancholia* are obscure, but in its first occurrence, in the writings of the Hippocratic school, its meaning, 'black-bile disease', is clear. Soon after this usage was established, its associations with the physical feelings of biliousness and cognitive or emotional darkness began to generate new metaphorical extensions. By the Renaissance there had developed an enormously rich and diverse range of tropes, symbols, and images connected with melancholia. The term *depression* has a very different history. It was not sanctioned by medical authority until quite late in its history. Until then its force derived purely from the descriptive aptness and metaphorical richness of the ideas of pressure and downwards motion. However, once Emil Kraepelin had installed *depression* as a head category, it possessed a sanction of authority that enabled it to dominate the discourse.

If melancholia required a particular scientific lens to make it objectively visible, the subjective experience of melancholia required self-consciousness. Here I am not talking about the experience of emotional and physical pain, which may be felt in quite un-self-conscious ways. The full spectrum of melancholic symptoms ranged from the purely physical through the emotional to the purely cognitive: stomach pains and general debility; emotional and affective malaise, such as a sadness akin to mourning; fear and paranoia; self-loathing and pessimism. I have argued that the symptoms at the cognitive end of the spectrum will occur most frequently in a culture that assigns a positive value to self-consciousness. We experience the florid psychological symptoms of melancholia because our culture encourages us to attend to the state of our inner life. Self-focused attention exacerbates the cognitive symptoms of the malaise and turns it into full-blown psychological melancholia. It gives fear and sadness a cognitive dimension, turning them into paranoia, self-loathing, and pessimism. Once these cognitive habits are established, they can take on a life of their own and they can cause the emotional pain, which might otherwise have ebbed away, to persist.

With its culturally variable cognitive content, the character of melancholia depends on social factors. Opponents of psychiatric realism have therefore argued that melancholia is socially constructed, and this presumably means it cannot qualify as a natural kind. A way through these arguments was outlined in the Introduction, and I shall refrain from repeating it here. How does the self-consciousness model add to the case for realism? The social factor that more than any other helps to create melancholia is a culturally sanctioned belief in the value of self-consciousness. Melancholia is socially constructed in the sense that it depends on the way our culture encourages us to focus on the self. By virtue of this, the self-consciousness model helps to overcome a difficulty in the history of melancholia. Like the other affective disorders, melancholia is highly cognitively penetrable. For instance, religious beliefs about sin and salvation have a powerful impact on melancholy feelings of low self-esteem. Obviously, then, melancholia must be highly sensitive to cultural change. However, if Jackson is right about the consistency of the core psychological symptoms of melancholia, it would appear that the psychological symptoms of melancholia have changed relatively little. And it hardly needs saying that the West has undergone deep and far-reaching cultural change since Hippocrates' time. The self-consciousness model goes some way towards solving this conundrum. It explains the durability of melancholia (in part at least) in terms of those cultural and intellectual values that have endured. Like our preference for a version of the Ionic method of science, our continuing focus on the self forms a robust and durable niche in which melancholia has been able to persist over the *longue durée*.

Gender furnishes another powerful antirealist argument. Some mental disorders come deeply gendered. A paradigmatic example is hysteria. Its very existence is predicated on socially constructed beliefs about the physical and emotional nature of women – that women are by nature less rational than men, and that women's bodies function properly only if regularly impregnated. Is melancholia as deeply gendered as hysteria, and does the gender argument undermine the case for the reality of melancholia? If it were to do so, it would have to show that gendering affects melancholia across a large part of its history in relatively consistent ways, so that melancholia as a whole could be shown to be socially constructed by beliefs about gender. However, this is not what we find. At particular times and places, melancholia is clearly gendered, but the gendering takes a large number of different and often contradictory forms. Moreover, melancholia is nowhere near as deeply gendered as hysteria. Indeed, we often find that melancholia itself is not gendered; rather, the gendering comes from neighbouring concepts such as physiological theories or the idea of genius. The evidence that melancholia is constructed at a fundamental level by a small number of enduring beliefs about women is weak.

The self-consciousness model helps us to avoid some of the pitfalls associated with other theories of melancholia. Most theories of melancholia have used social or economic models. The rise of early modern capitalism, the emergence of modern individualism, religious schism, and war – these have been offered as explanations for the supposed epidemic of early modern melancholia. An evident weakness of these models is that they are tied to specific places and times, even if the places and times have fairly broad parameters. Obviously, none of the models apply to the origins of melancholia in classical Greece or to late antiquity or to the golden age of Islamic culture in the Middle Ages. They also have difficulty in accounting for the peculiar diffusion of melancholia through the social strata. If the case for social or economic causation is going to be plausible, it would have to show that social groups are affected by melancholia broadly to the same extent as they are affected by social and economic change. But this appears not to be the case. Melancholia generally did not spread laterally across social strata; it infected pockets of the population, and these pockets were defined not socially but in terms of beliefs and ideologies (e.g. Puritanism). The self-consciousness model fits the historical data much better. The earliest evidence of melancholia in fifth-century BC Greece coincided with a well-attested upsurge of interest in self-examination. The same can be said of the 'golden ages' of melancholia in Renaissance Italy, Elizabethan and Jacobean England, and the European age of sensibility.

The geographical spread of melancholia was likewise determined by the diffusion of Western medical science and Western self-consciousness. The great non-Western cultures, no less 'advanced' than the West, have nothing to parallel melancholia. In most cases we find that the philosophical and religious cultures of, say, ancient and 'medieval' India and China viewed self-consciousness as something to be avoided. Consequently, the florid psychological symptoms of Western melancholia tended not to develop. If these philosophical and religious belief systems prevented melancholia from flourishing, one might even see them – Buddhism would be a prime example – as conferring some degree of protection against melancholia. No wonder that since the 1960s many in the West have seen Buddhism as a refuge from the Western malaise.

When we turn to the impact of melancholia on politics, philosophy, and the arts, the self-consciousness model comes into its own, because it allows melancholia to have meaningful cognitive content, unlike some other theories of melancholia. Most modern theories of melancholia have denied it any cognitive content. In his *Anthropology from a Pragmatic Point of View* (*Anthropologie in pragmatischer Hinsicht*, 1798), Kant drew a distinction between character and temperament. The former is a product of the will; it expresses the practical principles according to which a person behaves. It has cognitive content – it is, in Kant's terminology, a 'manner of thinking' ('Denkungsart'). The four temperaments, on the other hand, are pathological and have no cognitive or indeed moral content.[2] For Kant, therefore, melancholia is cognitively empty. However, if the self-consciousness model is correct, a large part of melancholic behaviour consists precisely in its cognitive content. This opens up the possibility that melancholia could be politically and philosophically meaningful. Admittedly, it might still be hard to find in melancholy philosophy or politics a fully worked out, positive programme. Still, melancholy cognition may yield meaningful forms of philosophical and political critique.

As for melancholia in the arts, the quantity of melancholy art, music, and literature is enormous and many times greater than the cultural uses of the sanguine, bilious, or choleric temperaments. In the last ten years there has been an upsurge in writing about the first-hand experience of depression, in memoirs, novels, and poetry. In the seventeenth and eighteenth centuries, similar quantities of writing about melancholia were produced. The sheer volume of material is extraordinary. The self-consciousness model accounts for this by locating melancholia at the heart of Western culture. On the view set out in these pages, melancholia is an affective disorder that develops florid psychological expressions, such as self-loathing, paranoia, obsessive rumination, and pessimism. These psychological expressions have flourished in milieus that encourage intense focus on inner experience. Such self-directed focus has been central to Western culture, intermittently at least, since the classical era in Ancient Greece. It comes as no surprise then that there has been so much melancholia in music, art, and especially literature.

Melancholy literature is not only ubiquitous; some of it is exceptionally rich and complex. Here again the self-consciousness model is helpful because it puts the emphasis on cognition rather than psychology. In Chapter 5, I argued that we should be cautious about attributing the quality of melancholy literature directly to the melancholy psychology of its authors. We simply do not know enough about the psychology of creativity to be able to say that Byron was a great poet because he suffered from bipolar disorder. Instead I proposed that melancholia offered

---

[2] Immanuel Kant, *Werke in zehn Bänden*, ed. Wilhelm Weischedel (Darmstadt: Wissenschaftliche Buchgesellschaft, 1983), vol. X, 633–4.

thinkers and writers what they believed to be real intellectual and artistic gains, and that this might explain the attractiveness of melancholia as a literary topos. The results of this philosophical and literary interest in melancholia are plain to see throughout the Western tradition. The evidence ranges from large-scale philosophical and aesthetic projects (e.g. Schiller's or T. S. Eliot's accounts of modern culture) to smaller-scale but widespread phenomena such as the powerful and enduring trope of the melancholic wandering in pathless wastes.

In the brief compass of this book it has not been possible to cover much of the material in detail. Most of my argument has been at a fairly high level of generality. One area in particular that needs to be worked out in detail is the idea of self-consciousness. I have avoided giving the idea of self-consciousness any philosophical depth and have preferred to use a fairly simple definition of self-consciousness from cognitive psychology. My reasons for doing so were partly a matter of competence: the philosophy of self-consciousness is not an area I feel competent to discuss. Some historically inclined sociologists, anthropologists, and philosophers have argued that melancholia might be connected with the rise of self-consciousness or (more often) individualism in the West. My concerns about these arguments are spelt out in Chapter 4. There is also a historiographical argument for keeping the idea of self-consciousness simple and flexible. In this way we can avoid committing ourselves to historically specific notions of self-consciousness that would limit the model's range of application. It may be that this worry is unjustified, and that there is a robust and flexible philosophical model of self-consciousness that would enrich the model.

The self-consciousness model is likely to face fairly stiff resistance in the cultural field. Much of the detailed work on literary melancholia has been from a psychoanalytical perspective. (Again for reasons of space I have not been able to give proper recognition to the wealth of psychoanalytical or indeed non-psychoanalytical literary criticism on melancholia.)[3] Melancholy politics has traditionally been read in terms of a cognitive deficit: the work of Shoshana Felman and Wolf Lepenies suggests that melancholia represents a failure or inability to engage in politics.[4] A similar move occurs in psychoanalytical readings of melancholy literature. One of the first principles of psychoanalysis is, after all,

---

[3] Fredric V. Bogel, *Literature and Insubstantiality in Later Eighteenth-Century England* (Princeton University Press, 1984); Schiesari, *The Gendering of Melancholia*; Lynn Enterline, *The Tears of Narcissus: Melancholia and Masculinity in Early Modern Writing* (Stanford University Press, 1995).

[4] Felman, *What Does a Woman Want?*, 21; Lepenies, *Melancholy and Society*, 61.

that cognitive content is not to be taken at face value. The self-consciousness model, by contrast, implies a determinedly cognitivist view of melancholia.

Many of the difficulties in understanding early modern melancholia stem from the idea that melancholia might be a fashionable pose for the idle courtier, the unhappy lover, or the poetic genius. I believe that the importance of fashionable melancholia has been overstated. The evidence for fashionable melancholia should not lead us to conclude that melancholia was inauthentic to any substantial extent. I suspect that the trope of the melancholy genius found in texts from Ficino to Shakespeare and on to Goethe has given the melancholy genius undue prominence. Cultural histories of melancholia have not helped. The great work of Raymond Klibansky, Erwin Panofsky, and Fritz Saxl, *Saturn and Melancholy*, which traces the tradition of the melancholy genius up to Dürer's *Melencolia I*, has been by far the most influential modern account of melancholia. It could be argued that the self-consciousness model also risks giving this tradition undue prominence. If melancholia is so closely bound up with self-consciousness, must it not perforce seem inauthentic and easy to fabricate? We do not ordinarily worry about the question of authenticity even in highly self-conscious mental disorders. Suicidal behaviour is manifestly self-conscious, and that does not make it any less symptomatic of a mental disorder. Even suicidal behaviour that seems to contain an act of communication – what we commonly and misleadingly refer to as a 'cry for help' – still counts as clinically significant. In cases like this, most people would conclude that self-consciousness is compatible with authenticity. At the same time it has to be admitted that suicide and self-harm have become cultural markers for certain groups of young people. In her memoir of depression, *Prozac Nation* (1994), Elizabeth Wurtzel observes that the grunge and goth subcultures that emerged out of the alternative music scene of the mid 1980s lent a dangerous glamour to suicidal and depressive behaviour.[5] But should the fact that suicide and depression have been imitated in popular music incline us to scepticism about the clinical phenomena? Certainly not. I would contend that taking Dürer's *Melencholia I* or Shakespeare's *Hamlet* as paradigms of early modern melancholia is not that different from trying to understand depression today through Seattle grunge music. It risks ignoring or trivializing a vast hinterland of ordinary, unglamorous pain.

Fashionable melancholia may have been a minority phenomenon, and its significance within the history of melancholia may have been exaggerated, but there can be little doubt that it happened. Some early modern

---

[5] Elizabeth Wurtzel, *Prozac Nation: Young and Depressed in America*, 2nd edn (London: Quartet Books, 1996), 307–11.

Europeans evidently adopted melancholic behaviour without experiencing any symptoms of a melancholic disorder. Elizabethan men stood with their arms crossed, wore black and dishevelled clothing, and pulled their hats down over their eyes. Eighteenth-century men (and increasingly women) cried and languished, improvised wistfully on the piano, and frequented graveyards – or at least they wrote about doing so. In cases like these, inauthentic forms of melancholia are easy enough to spot. Some cases are less clear. Is Hamlet genuinely melancholic? Or Werther? To some extent the question whether they were really melancholic is misguided, as Hamlet and Werther are fictional characters. Were there any real cases like Werther and Hamlet – people whose melancholia seemed to sit uneasily between illness and fashion? The self-consciousness model suggests there probably were. There are likely to have been people who were not truly melancholic but appeared to be so. (I read Hamlet as a representation of this type.) Melancholic behaviour was so cognitively penetrable, so permeated by cultural norms, that it was possible to ape melancholia, and for a character like Hamlet it made sense to do so. Equally, there are likely to have been authentic melancholics who looked like fakes because they showed such a strong awareness of the culturally conditioned forms of their behaviour and because their melancholia extended so far into the realm of cultural production. Werther can be read in this way. The self-consciousness model helps to explain how such an intractable grey area of real-life Hamlets and Werthers might have come about. Nonetheless, the dichotomy of authenticity and inauthenticity still exists; the realism about melancholia that partners the self-consciousness model obliges us to discriminate between the authentic and inauthentic melancholics.

Questions remain about the psychological and social reasons for melancholy behaviour. What psychological and social sense does it make to behave in these ways? How does it benefit a melancholic (or indeed non-melancholic) to engage in the typical melancholy behaviour? It may be that melancholy behaviour serves to release uncomfortable pent-up energy or to externalize emotional pain. This might in turn explain the conundrum of pleasurable or 'white' melancholia. It may be that engagement in cultural activities with melancholia as their theme has offered some people a form of relief by enabling them to externalize their suffering. But this is a rather simplistic answer, and more (and more sophisticated) work would be needed here. As for social reasons for melancholy behaviour, we have seen that in the eighteenth century melancholia offered a mode of behaviour that felt right to people who found themselves excluded from economic progress. It is tempting here to draw a parallel with the depressive and suicidal behaviour of modern youth subcultures. In early modern melancholia a similar subcultural tribalism or identity politics might have been at work. Melancholy behaviour might have been a means for people to identify themselves as belonging to a group that was alienated from social norms.

For those people who made a significant investment in the culture of melancholia, whether they were authentically melancholy or not, I am inclined to give more weight to the arguments set out in Chapter 5. Evidently, some writers believed that writing from a stance of melancholia conferred intellectual or aesthetic advantages. These advantages led some people to adopt melancholy behaviour even if they had no immediate psychological or social compulsion to do so. On the cognitive side, melancholy behaviour seemed to confer the advantage of deep insight into the miserable or terrifying nature of reality. (Whether the melancholy image of reality was in fact more accurate is another matter; the analogy of the depressive realism hypothesis suggests a way in which it might at least have appeared so.) On the social side, melancholy behaviour had a natural fit with Western cultures of self-consciousness. In contexts where self-consciousness was esteemed, melancholia enjoyed high status, because it elevated self-consciousness to an extreme pitch. The hugely enthusiastic reception of Goethe's *Werther* testifies to the allure of melancholy self-consciousness: the novel gave its already highly self-conscious readers the impression of an even more heightened sense of self. And insofar as modes of self-consciousness competed with one another in the cultural sphere, and insofar as their exponents claimed to find greater existential intensity in one mode of self-consciousness than in another, adopting an intensely self-conscious melancholia might have been a way to trump other, less extreme forms of self-consciousness. For its fans *Werther* quite simply trumped all other available modes of representing and thinking about the self.

Werther was one of the best-selling novels of the late eighteenth century, though the lack of a copyright law in Germany meant that pirate publishers did better out of the novel than Goethe himself. For Goethe the less tangible rewards of public recognition were to prove more important. He was the first German writer in the eighteenth century to win European fame, thanks to *Werther*. At the Congress of Erfurt in 1808, Napoleon requested a meeting with Goethe, not because of Goethe's diplomatic role at the congress, but because he was the author of *Werther*. According to one report, Napoleon ended their conversation with the words 'Voilà un homme!'[6] The award of the Légion d'honneur followed. All for a short novel about a young melancholic who killed himself.

---

[6] Johann Wolfgang von Goethe, *Sämtliche Werke nach Epochen seines Schaffens*, ed. Karl Richer *et al.*, 21 vols. in 33 (Munich: Hanser, 1985–1999), vol. XIV, 850.

Western culture accords high status to virtuosi in self-consciousness. We honour those who mine the depths of the self. And if the depths of the self turn out to be complex and intractable, the rewards for laying them bare will be all the greater. Discovery bleeds into invention. Such are the rewards for virtuosity in self-consciousness that it may be tempting to create complexity and intractability where none exists. In the words of Jean Kerr: 'Some people have such a talent for making the best of a bad situation that they go around creating bad situations so they can make the best of them.'[7] Are melancholics like this? Definitely yes and no.

---

[7] The lines are spoken by the character Mary in Jean Kerr, *Mary, Mary* (London: Samuel French, 1963), 57.

Bibliography

Aiken, Conrad, 'An Anatomy of Melancholy', *Sewanee Review* 74 (1966), 188–96.

Allan, Lorraine G., Shepard Siegel, and Samuel Hannah, 'The Sad Truth About Depressive Realism', *Quarterly Journal of Experimental Psychology* 60 (2007), 482–95.

Alloy, Lauren B., and Lyn Y. Abramson, 'Depressive Realism: Four Theoretical Perspectives', in Lauren B. Alloy (ed.), *Cognitive Processes in Depression* (New York: Guilford Press, 1988), 223–65.

Alloy, Lauren B., and Alan J. Lipman, 'Depression and Selection of Positive and Negative Social Feedback: Motivated Preference or Cognitive Balance?', *Journal of Abnormal Psychology* 101 (1992), 310–13.

Amabile, T. M., 'Motivation and Creativity: Effects of Motivational Orientation on Creative Writers', *Journal of Personality and Social Psychology* 48 (1985), 393–7.

American Psychiatric Association, *Diagnostic and Statistical Manual of Mental Disorders*, 3rd edn (DSM-III) (Washington, DC: APA, 1980).

Diagnostic and Statistical Manual of Mental Disorders, 4th edn; text rev. (DSM-IV-TR) (Washington, DC: APA, 2000).

Diagnostic and Statistical Manual of Mental Disorders, 5th edn (DSM-5) (Arlington, VA: APA, 2013).

Anon., *An Essay on the Nature, Use, and Abuse, of Tea, in a Letter to a Lady; With an Account of its Mechanical Operation* (London: Bettenham, 1722).

Appignanesi, Lisa, *Mad, Bad and Sad: A History of Women and the Mind Doctors from 1800* (London: Virago, 2009).

Arctinus of Miletus [attrib.], *Sack of Ilion*, in *Greek Epic Fragments*, ed. and trans. M. L. West, Loeb Classical Library (Cambridge, MA: Harvard University Press, 2003).

Arikha, Noga, *Passions and Tempers: A History of the Humours* (New York: Ecco, 2007).

Aristotle, *The Complete Works of Aristotle. The Revised Oxford Translation*, ed. Jonathan Barnes, 2 vols., Bollingen Series LXXI (Princeton University Press, 1984).

Problems, trans. W. H. Hett, Loeb Classical Library, 2 vols. (Cambridge, MA: Harvard University Press, 1936–7).

Baas, Matthijs, Carsten K. W. De Dreu, and Bernard A. Nijstad, 'A Meta-Analysis of 25 Years of Mood–Creativity Research: Hedonic Tone, Activation, or Regulatory Focus?', *Psychological Bulletin* 134 (2008), 779–806.

Baker, D., and H. Taylor, 'The Relation Between Condition-Specific Morbidity, Social Support and Material Deprivation in Pregnancy and Early Motherhood', *Social Science and Medicine* 45 (1997), 1325–36.

Barker-Benfield, G. J., *The Culture of Sensibility: Sex and Society in Eighteenth-Century Britain* (University of Chicago Press, 1992).

Barton, Anne, 'Introduction', in William Shakespeare, *Hamlet*, The New Penguin Shakespeare, ed. T. J. B. Spencer (London: Penguin, 1980), 7–54.

Beck, Aaron T., *Cognitive Therapy and the Emotional Disorders* (Harmondsworth: Penguin, 1989).

Beecher, Donald A., 'From Myth to Narrative: Saturn in Lefevre and Caxton', in *Saturn from Antiquity to the Renaissance* (University of Toronto Italian Studies 8), ed. Massimo Ciavolella and Amilcare A. Iannucci (Ottawa: Dovehouse, 1992), 79–90.

Begemann, Christian, *Furcht und Angst im Prozeß der Aufklärung: zu Literatur und Bewußtseinsgeschichte des 18. Jahrhunderts* (Frankfurt/Main: Athenäum, 1987).

Bell, Matthew, *The German Tradition of Psychology in Literature and Thought, 1700–1840* (Cambridge University Press, 2005).

Bentall, Richard P., *Madness Explained: Psychosis and Human Nature* (Harmondsworth: Penguin, 2004).

Berkeley, George, *The Works of George Berkeley, DD, Late Bishop of Cloyne in Ireland: To which is Added an Account of his Life, and Several of his Letters* (Dublin: Exshaw, 1784).

Blair, Hugh, *Critical Dissertation on the Poems of Ossian* (London: Becket and De Hondt, 1763).

Bloor, David, *Knowledge and Social Imagery* (London: Routledge & Kegan Paul, 1976).

Boase, Roger, *The Origin and Meaning of Courtly Love: A Critical Study of European Scholarship* (Manchester University Press, 1977).

Boerhaave, Herman, *Practical Aphorisms* (London: Cowse, 1715).

Boesch, Christophe, *Wild Cultures: A Comparison Between Chimpanzee and Human Cultures* (Cambridge University Press, 2012).

Bogel, Fredric V., *Literature and Insubstantiality in Later Eighteenth-Century England* (Princeton University Press, 1984).

Boghossian, Paul A., 'What Is Social Construction?', *Times Literary Supplement* 5108 (23 February 2001), 6–8.

Borch-Jacobsen, Mikkel, *Making Minds and Madness: From Hysteria to Depression* (Cambridge University Press, 2009).

Boyd, Richard, 'Realism, Anti-Foundationalism and the Enthusiasm for Natural Kinds', *Philosophical Studies* 61 (1991), 127–48.

'Homeostasis, Species, and Higher Taxa', in Robert A. Wilson (ed.), *Species: New Interdisciplinary Essays* (Cambridge, MA: MIT Press, 1999), 141–85.

Bunke, Simon, *Heimweh. Studien zur Kultur- und Literaturgeschichte einer tödlichen Krankheit* (Freiburg: Rombach, 2009).

Burckhardt, Jacob, *The Civilization of the Renaissance in Italy* (Harmondsworth: Penguin, 1990).

The Greeks and Greek Civilization (New York: St Martin's Press, 1998).

Burton, Robert, *The Anatomy of Melancholy*, ed. Thomas C. Faulkner *et al.*, 5 vols. (Oxford University Press, 1989).

Byron, George Gordon, Lord, *Works. Poetry*, vol. VI, ed. Ernest Hartley Coleridge (London: Murray, 1905).

Bywater, Michael, *Lost Worlds: What Have We Lost, and Where Did It Go?* (Cambridge: Granta, 2004).

Carothers, J. C., 'Frontal Lobe Function and the African', *Journal of Mental Sciences* 97 (1951), 12–48.

Cheyne, George, *An Essay of Health and Long Life* (Dublin: Wilmot, 1725).

The English Malady, ed. Roy Porter (London: Routledge, 1991).

Colvin, C. Randall, and Jack Block, 'Do Positive Illusions Foster Mental Health? An Examination of the Taylor and Brown Formulation', *Psychological Bulletin* 116 (1994), 3–20.

Cooper, J. E., *et al.*, *Psychiatric Diagnosis in New York and London* (Oxford University Press, 1972).

Cooper, Rachel, 'Why Hacking Is Wrong About Human Kinds', *British Journal of the Philosophy of Science* 55 (2004), 73–85.

Cosmides, Leda, and John Tooby, 'Toward an Evolutionary Taxonomy of Treatable Conditions', *Journal of Abnormal Psychology* 108 (1999), 453–64.

Crichton, Alexander, *An Inquiry into the Nature and Origin of Mental Derangement*, 2 vols. (London: T. Cadell, W. Davies, 1798).

Cullen, William, *Lectures on the Materia Medica* (London: Lowndes, 1773).

Dalley, Stephanie (ed.), *Myths from Mesopotamia: Creation, the Flood, Gilgamesh, and Others* (Oxford University Press, 1989).

Damrau, Peter, *The Reception of English Puritan Literature in Germany* (London: Maney, 2006).

Darwin, Charles, *The Expression of the Emotions in Man and Animals*, ed. Paul Ekman (London: HarperCollins, 1998).

Dawkins, Richard, *The Extended Phenotype: The Long Reach of the Gene* (Oxford University Press, 1999).

Depression: Treatment and Management of Depression in Adults, Including Adults with a Chronic Physical Health Problem, CG90 and 91 (London: National Institute for Health and Clinical Excellence, 2009).

Descartes, Réné, *The Philosophical Writings of Descartes*, trans. John Cottingham, Robert Stoothoff, and Dugald Murdoch, 3 vols. (Cambridge University Press, 1984–91).

Diderot, Denis, and Jean le Rond d'Alembert (eds.), *Encyclopédie, ou Dictionnaire raisonné des sciences, des arts et des métiers* (Paris: Briasson *et al.*, 1751–72).

Dienstag, Joshua Foa, *Pessimism: Philosophy, Ethic, Spirit* (Princeton University Press, 2006).

Dobson, Keith S., and Dennis Pusch, 'A Test of the Depressive Realism Hypothesis in Clinically Depressed Subjects', *Cognitive Therapy and Research* 19 (1995), 179–94.

Dobson, William, Letter to Sir Hans Sloane, 12 September 1730, London, British Library, MS Sloane 4075, fol. 79.

Dols, Michael W., *Majnūn: The Madman in Islamic Society* (Oxford University Press, 1992).

Dooley, D., R. Catalano, and G. Wilson, 'Depression and Unemployment: Panel Findings from the Epidemiologic Catchment Area study', *American Journal of Community Psychology* 22 (1994), 745–65.

Du Laurens, André, *A Discourse of the Preservation of the Sight: of Melancholike Diseases; of Rheumes, and of Old Age* (London: Kingston, 1599).

Dupré, John, *The Disorder of Things: Metaphysical Foundations of the Disunity of Science* (Cambridge, MA: Harvard University Press, 1993).

'Natural Kinds and Biological Taxa', *Philosophical Review* 90 (1981), 66–90.

Dykman, Benjamin M., *et al.*, 'Processing of Ambiguous and Unambiguous Feedback by Depressed and Nondepressed College Students: Schematic Biases and Their Implications for Depressive Realism', *Journal of Personal and Social Psychology* 56 (1989), 431–45.

Edgerton, Robert B., 'Conceptions of Psychosis in East-African Societies', in David Landy (ed.), *Culture, Disease and Healing: Studies in Medical Anthropology* (New York: Macmillan, 1977).

Ehrenreich, Barbara, *Dancing in the Streets: A History of Collective Joy* (London: Granta, 2007).

Ekman, Paul, *Emotions Revealed: Understanding Faces and Feelings* (London: Weidenfeld & Nicholson, 2003).

Eliot, T. S., *Collected Poems 1909–1935* (London: Faber & Faber, 1936).

Ellis, Markman, *The Politics of Sensibility: Race, Gender and Commerce in the Sentimental Novel* (Cambridge University Press, 1996).

Elyot, Thomas, *The Castel of Helthe* (London: Berthelet, 1539).

Enterline, Lynn, *The Tears of Narcissus: Melancholia and Masculinity in Early Modern Writing* (Stanford University Press, 1995).

Evans, R. J. W., *Rudolf II and His World: A Study in Intellectual History, 1576–1612* (Oxford University Press, 1973).

Farrington, Benjamin, *Greek Science* (Nottingham: Spokesman, 1980).

Felman, Shoshana, *What Does a Woman Want? Reading and Sexual Difference* (Baltimore, MD: Johns Hopkins University Press, 1993).

Ferrand, Jacques, *A Treatise on Lovesickness*, trans. and ed. by Donald A. Beecher and Massimo Ciavolella (Syracuse, NY: Syracuse University Press, 1990).

Ficino, Marsilio, *The Book of Life*, trans. Charles Boer (Woodstock, CT: Spring, 1994).

Finch, Anne, *The Poems of Anne, Countess of Winchilsea*, ed. by Myra Reynolds (University of Chicago Press, 1903).

Flashar, Helmut, *Melancholie und Melancholiker in den medizinischen Theorien der Antike* (Berlin: de Gruyter, 1966).

Flemming, Rebecca, *Medicine and the Making of Roman Women: Gender, Nature and Authority from Celsus to Galen* (Oxford University Press, 2000).

Foucault, Michel, *History of Madness* (London: Routledge, 2006).

Freud, Sigmund, 'Mourning and Melancholia', in Freud, *On Murder, Mourning and Melancholia*, trans. Shaun Whiteside (London: Penguin, 2005), 201–18.

Fromm, Erich, *Fear of Freedom* (London: Routledge, 2001).

Fumaroli, Marc, 'La Mélancolie et ses remèdes. Classicisme français et maladie de l'âme', in Fumaroli, *La Diplomatie de l'esprit. De Montaigne à La Fontaine* (Paris: Hermann, 1994), 403–39.

Galen, *Opera Omnia*, ed. C. G. Kühn, 20 vols. (Leipzig: Knobloch, 1821–33).

Goethe, Johann Wolfgang von, *Sämtliche Werke nach Epochen seines Schaffens*, ed. Karl Richer *et al.*, 21 vols. in 33 (Munich: Hanser, 1985–1999).

Selected Poems, trans. John Whaley (London: J. M. Dent, 1998).

The Sorrows of Young Werther, trans. Michael Hulse (Harmondsworth: Penguin, 1989).

Werke, ed. Erich Schmidt *et al.*, 146 vols. (Weimar: Böhlau, 1887–1919).

Goldsmith, Oliver, *Collected Works of Oliver Goldsmith*, ed. Arther Friedman, 5 vols. (Oxford University Press, 1966).

Golin, Sanford, *et al.*, 'The Illusion of Control Among Depressed Patients', *Journal of Abnormal Psychology* 88 (1979), 454–7.

Golin, Sanford, Francis Terrell, and Barbara Johnson, 'Depression and the Illusion of Control', *Journal of Abnormal Psychology* 86 (1977), 440–2.

Gomm, R., 'Mental Health and Inequality' in *Mental Health Matters – A Reader*, ed. T. Heller *et al.* (Basingstoke: Open University Press, 1996), 110–20.

Gowland, Angus, 'The Ethics of Renaissance Melancholy', *Intellectual History Review* 18 (2008), 103–17.

'The Problem of Early Modern Melancholy', *Past and Present* 191 (2006), 77–120.

The Worlds of Renaissance Melancholy: Robert Burton in Context (New York: Cambridge University Press, 2006).

Green, Thomas, *A Dissertation on Enthusiasm; Shewing the Danger of its Late Increase, and the Great Mischiefs it has Occasioned, both in Ancient and Modern Times* (London: Oliver, 1755).

Gregory, John, *Elements of the Practice of Physic* (Edinburgh: Balfour and Smellie, 1788).

Griffiths, Paul, *What Emotions Really Are: The Problem of Psychological Categories* (University of Chicago Press, 1997).

Guimaraes, Livia, 'A Melancholy Skeptic', *Kriterion: Revista de Filosofia* 108 (2003), 180–90.

Hacking, Ian, *Mad Travellers: Reflections on the Reality of Transient Mental Illness* (Charlottesville, VA: University Press of Virginia, 1998).

Rewriting the Soul: Multiple Personality and the Sciences of Memory (Princeton University Press, 1995).

The Social Construction of What? (Cambridge, MA: Harvard University Press, 1999).

Haller, Albrecht von, *First Lines of Physiology*, 2 vols. (Edinburgh: Elliot, 1786).

Happé, Francesca, 'Autism: Cognitive Deficit or Cognitive Style?', *Trends in Cognitive Sciences* 3 (1999), 216–22.

Harmer, Thomas, *The Good Liable to Intellectual Disorders, of the Melancholy Kind, Equally with Others: A Sermon* (London: Hawes, 1779).

Healy, David, *The Antidepressant Era* (Cambridge, MA: Harvard University Press, 1997).

Heffernan, Carol Falvo, *The Melancholy Muse: Chaucer, Shakespeare, and Early Medicine* (Pittsburgh, PA: Duquesne University Press, 1995).

Helvétius, Claude-Adrien, *Œuvres* (Paris: Didot l'aîné, 1795).

Heyd, Michael, 'The Reaction to Enthusiasm', *Journal of Modern History* 53 (1981), 258–80.

Hildegard of Bingen, *On Natural Philosophy and Medicine*, ed. and trans. Margret Berger (Cambridge: Brewer, 1999).

Hippocrates, *Hippocrates I*, trans. W. H. S. Jones, Loeb Classical Library (London: Heinemann, 1948).

Hippocrates IV, trans. W. H. S. Jones, Loeb Classical Library (London: Heinemann, 1979).

Hippocrates VII, trans. Wesley D. Smith, Loeb Classical Library (Cambridge, MA: Harvard University Press, 1975).

Opera, ed. Hugo Kuehlewein (Leipzig: Teubner, 1894–1902).

Hoffmann, Friedrich, *A System of the Practice of Medicine*, 2 vols. (London: Murray, 1783).

Hofmannsthal, Hugo von, *The Whole Difference: Selected Writings of Hugo von Hofmannsthal*, ed. J. D. McClatchy (Princeton University Press, 2008).

Hopton, J. L., and S. M. Hunt, 'Housing Conditions and Mental Health in a Disadvantaged Area in Scotland', *Journal of Epidemiology and Community Health* 50 (1996), 56–61.

Hugo, Victor, *Œuvres Poétiques*, ed. Pierre Albouy, 3 vols. (Paris: Gallimard, 1964–74).

Hull, David L., 'The Effect of Essentialism on Taxonomy – Two Thousand Years of Stasis', *British Journal for the Philosophy of Science* 15 (1965), 314–26, and 16 (1965), 1–18.

Hume, David, *Essays Moral, Political, and Literary*, 4 vols. (London: Millar, 1760).

The Letters of David Hume, ed. J. Y. T. Greig, 2 vols. (Oxford University Press, 1932).

Principal Writings on Religion including 'Dialogues Concerning Natural Religion' and 'Natural History of Religion', ed. J. C. A. Gaskin (Oxford University Press, 1993).

A Treatise of Human Nature, ed. L. A. Selby-Bigge, rev. P. H. Nidditch (Oxford University Press, 1978).

Ibn 'Imrān, Isḥāq, *Maqāla fī'l-mālīḫūliyā (Abhandlung über die Melancholie)* and Constantinus Africanus, *Libri duo de melancholia*, ed. and trans. Karl Garbers (Hamburg: Buske, 1977).

Ingram, Rick E., 'Self-Focused Attention in Clinical Disorders: Review and a Conceptual Model', *Psychological Bulletin* 107 (1990), 156–76.

Inwood, Brad, and Pierluigi Donini, 'Stoic Ethics', *The Cambridge History of Hellenistic Philosophy*, ed. Keimpe Algra *et al.* (Cambridge University Press, 1999), 675–738.

Jackson, Stanley, 'Galen – On Mental Disorders', *Journal of the History of the Behavioral Sciences* 5 (1969), 365–84.

Melancholia and Depression: From Hippocratic Times to Modern Times (New Haven, CT: Yale University Press, 1986).

'Melancholia and the Waning of the Humoral Theory', *Journal of the History of Medicine* 33 (1978), 367–76.

Jamison, Kay Redfield, *Touched with Fire: Manic-Depressive Illness and the Artistic Temperament* (New York: Free Press, 1993).

Johnson, Samuel, *A Dictionary of the English Language: In which the Words are Deduced from their Originals, and Illustrated in their Different Significations, by*

Examples from the Best Writers, to which are Prefixed a History of the Language, and an English Grammar, 2 vols. (London: Strahan, 1755–6).

Jouanna, Jacques, 'At the Roots of Melancholy: Is Greek Medicine Melancholic?', in Jouanna, *Greek Medicine from Hippocrates to Galen: Selected Papers* (Leiden; Boston: Brill, 2012), 229–60.

Kant, Immanuel, *Werke in zehn Bänden*, ed. Wilhelm Weischedel (Darmstadt: Wissenschaftliche Buchgesellschaft, 1983).

Keats, John, *Poetical Works*, ed. H. W. Garrod (Oxford University Press, 1989).

Kerr, Jean, *Mary, Mary* (London: Samuel French, 1963).

Kessler, R. C., C. Nelson, K. A. McGonagle, *et al.*, 'Comorbidity of DSM-III-R Major Depressive Disorder in the General Population: Results from the US National Comorbidity Survey', *British Journal of Psychiatry* 168, suppl. 30 (1996), 17–30.

Khalidi, Muhammad Ali, 'Interactive Kinds', *British Journal for the Philosophy of Science* 61 (2010), 335–60.

Kierkegaard, Søren, *The Concept of Anxiety*, trans. Reidar Thomte (Princeton University Press, 1980).

King, John, *An Essay on Hot and Cold Bathing* (London: Bettenham, 1737).

King, John Owen, III, *The Iron of Melancholy: Structures of Spiritual Conversion from the Puritan Conscience to Victorian Neurosis* (Middletown, CT: Wesleyan University Press, 1983).

Kirsch, Irving, *The Emperor's New Drugs: Exploding the Antidepressant Myth* (London: The Bodley Head, 2009).

Kleinman, Arthur, *Social Origins of Distress and Disease: Depression, Neurasthesia and Pain in Modern China* (Newhaven, CT: Yale University Press, 1988).

Klibansky, Raymond, Erwin Panofsky, and Fritz Saxl, *Saturn and Melancholy: Studies in the History of Natural Philosophy, Religion, and Art* (New York: Basic Books, 1964).

Knights, L. C., 'Seventeenth-Century Melancholy', *Criterion* 13 (1933–4), 97–112.

Konstan, David, *A Life Worthy of the Gods: The Materialist Psychology of Epicurus* (Las Vegas, NV: Parmenides, 2008).

Kraepelin, Emil, *Psychiatry: A Textbook for Students and Physicians*, 6th edn, reprint (Canton, MA: Science History Publications, 1990).

Kuhn, Thomas S., *The Structure of Scientific Revolutions* (University of Chicago Press, 1962).

Kutzer, Michael, *Anatomie des Wahnsinns: Geisteskrankheit im medizinischen Denken der frühen Neuzeit und die Anfänge der pathologischen Anatomie* (Hürtgenwald: Pressler, 1998).

Langhorne, J., 'Memoirs of the Author', in *The Poetical Works of Mr William Collins. With Memoirs of the Author; and Observations on his Genius and Writings* (London: Becket, 1771).

Layte, Richard, 'The Association Between Income Inequality and Mental Health: Testing Status Anxiety, Social Capital, and Neo-Materialist Explanations', *European Sociological Review* 28 (2011), 498–511.

Leader, Darian, *The New Black: Mourning, Melancholia and Depression* (London: Hamish Hamilton, 2008).

Leerssen, Joep, 'Sublime Landscape and National Character', in Gisela Holfter, Marieke Krajenbrink, and Edward Moxon-Browne (eds.), *Beziehungen und Identitäten: Österreich, Irland und die Schweiz* (Bern: Lang, 2004), 25–35.

Leibbrand-Wettley, Annemarie, 'Zur Psychopathologie und Dämonoligie bei Paracelsus und Johannes Weyer', in Joseph Schumacher, unter Mitarbeit von Martin Schrenk and Jörn Henning Wolf (eds.), *Melemata: Festschrift für Werner Leibbrand zum siebzigsten Geburtstag* (Mannheimer Großdruckerei, 1967), 65–73.

Lemmens, Willem, 'Melancholy of the Philosopher: Hume and Spinoza on Emotions and Wisdom', *Journal of Scottish Philosophy* 3 (2005), 47–65.

Lepenies, Wolf, *Melancholy and Society* (Cambridge, MA: Harvard University Press, 1992).

Lewis, G., *et al.*, 'Socioeconomic Status, Standard of Living, and Neurotic Disorder', *Lancet* 352 (1998), 605–9.

Liddell, Henry George, and Robert Scott, *A Greek-English Lexicon* (Oxford University Press, 1996).

Lloyd, G. E. R., *Early Greek Science: Thales to Aristotle* (London: Chatto & Windus, 1970).

  Magic, Reason and Experience: Studies in the Origin and Development of Greek Science (Cambridge University Press, 1979).

Lloyd, G. E. R., and Nathan Sivin, *The Way and the Word: Science and Medicine in Early China and Greece* (New Haven, CT: Yale University Press, 2002).

Lombros, César [Lombroso, Cesare], *L'Homme de génie* (Paris: Schleicher, 1889).

Ludwig, Arnold M., *The Price of Greatness: Resolving the Creativity and Madness Controversy* (New York: Guilford Press, 1995).

Luttwak, Edward, *Turbo-Capitalism: Winners and Losers in the Global Economy* (New York: HarperCollins, 1999).

Lutz, Catherine, 'Depression and the Translation of Emotional Worlds', in Arthur Kleinman and Byron Good (eds.), *Culture and Depression* (Berkeley, CA: University of California Press, 1985), 63–100.

Lynch, John W., George A. Kaplan, and Sarah J. Shema, 'Cumulative Impact of Sustained Economic Hardship on Physical, Cognitive, Psychological, and Social Functioning', *New England Journal of Medicine* 337 (1997), 1889–95.

MacCabe, James H., *et al.*, 'Excellent School Performance at Age 16 and Risk of Adult Bipolar Disorder: National Cohort Study', *British Journal of Psychology* 196 (2010), 109–15.

MacCulloch, Diarmaid, *The Reformation* (New York: Viking, 2004).

MacDonald, Michael, *Mystical Bedlam: Madness, Anxiety, and Healing in Seventeenth-Century England* (Cambridge University Press, 1981), 35.

MacKenzie, Henry, *The Man of Feeling* (Oxford University Press, 2001).

MacKenzie Matthew, 'Self-Awareness Without a Self: Buddhism and the Reflexivity of Awareness', *Asian Philosophy* 18 (2008), 245–66.

Maclean, Ian, *The Renaissance Notion of Woman: A Study in the Fortunes of Scholasticism and Medical Science in European Intellectual Life* (Cambridge University Press, 1980).

McAlindon, Thomas, *Shakespeare's Tragic Cosmos* (Cambridge University Press, 1996).

McEvilley, Thomas, *The Shape of Ancient Thought: Comparative Studies in Greek and Indian Philosophies* (New York: Allworth Press, 2002).

McKinsey, Michael, 'Anti-Individualism and Privileged Access', *Analysis* 51 (1991), 9–16.

McNally, Richard J., *What Is Mental Illness?* (Cambridge, MA: Harvard University Press, 2011).

Meltzer, H., *et al.*, *The Prevalence of Psychiatric Morbidity Among Adults Living in Private Households* (London: OPCS, 1995).

Midelfort, H. C. Erik, *A History of Madness in Sixteenth-Century Germany* (Stanford University Press, 1999).

Mad Princes of Renaissance Germany (Charlottesville, VA: University Press of Virginia, 1994).

Mio, Jeffrey Scott, *et al.* (eds.), *Key Words in Multicultural Interventions: A Dictionary* (Westport, CT; London: Greenwood, 1999).

Möbius, Paul Julius, 'Über das Studium der Talente', *Zeitschrift für Hypnotismus* 10 (1902), 66–74.

Montgomery, S. M., *et al.*, 'Unemployment Predates Symptoms of Depression and Anxiety Resulting in Medical Consultation in Young Men', *International Journal of Epidemiology* 28 (1999), 95–100.

Moreau, Jacques-Joseph, *La Psychologie morbide dans ses rapports avec la philosophie de l'histoire, ou De l'influence des névropathies sur le dynamisme intellectuel* (Paris: Masson, 1859).

Morris, Colin, *The Discovery of the Individual, 1050–1200* (University of Toronto Press, 1991).

Msetfi, Rachel M., *et al.*, 'Depressive Realism and Outcome Density Bias in Contingency Judgments: The Effect of the Context and Intertrial Interval', *Journal of Experimental Psychology. General* 134 (2005), 10–22.

Msetfi, Rachel M., Robin A. Murphy, and Jane Simpson, 'Depressive Realism and the Effect of Intertrial Interval on Judgements of Zero, Positive, and Negative Contingencies', *Quarterly Journal of Experimental Psychology* 60 (2007), 461–81.

Murphy, Dominic, *Psychiatry in the Scientific Image* (Cambridge, MA: MIT Press, 2006).

Nelson, R. E., and W. E. Craighead, 'Selective Recall of Positive and Negative Feedback, Self-Control Behaviors and Depression', *Journal of Abnormal Psychology* 86 (1977), 379–88.

Nolen-Hoeksema, Susan, 'Responses to Depression and Their Effects on the Duration of Depressive Episodes', *Journal of Abnormal Psychology* 100 (1991), 569–82.

Sex Differences in Depression (Stanford University Press, 1990).

Nutton, Vivian, *Ancient Medicine* (London: Routledge, 2004).

Olfson, M., B. Fireman, M. M. Weissman, *et al.*, 'Mental Disorders and Disability Among Patients in a Primary Care Group Practice', *American Journal of Psychiatry* 154 (1997), 1734–40.

Olson, Krista K., and LaDonna Pavetti, 'Personal and Family Challenges to the Successful Transition from Welfare to Work' (www.urban.org/publications/406850.html).

Opler, Marvin K., and S. Mouchly Small, 'Cultural Variables Affecting Somatic Complaints and Depression', *Psychosomatics: Journal of Consultation and Liaison Psychiatry* 9 (1968), 261–6.

Oquendo, Maria, Ewald Horwath, and Abigail Martinez, 'Ataques de Nervios: Proposed Diagnostic Criteria for a Culture-Specific Syndrome', *Culture, Medicine and Psychiatry* 16 (1992), 367–76.

Pacini, Rosemary, Francisco Muir, and Seymour Epstein, 'Depressive Realism from the Perspective of Cognitive-Experiential Self-Theory', *Journal of Personality and Social Psychology* 74 (1998), 1056–68.

Parker, Gordon, 'Editorial: Commentary on Diagnosing Major Depressive Disorder', *Journal of Nervous and Mental Disease* 194 (2006), 155–7.

Parker, Gordon, *et al.*, 'Issues for DSM-5: Whither Melancholia? The Case for Its Classification as a Distinct Mood Disorder', *American Journal of Psychiatry* 167 (2010), 745–7.

Parker, Seymour, 'Eskimo Psychopathology in the Context of Eskimo Personality and Culture', *American Anthropologist* 64 (1962), 76–96.

Perfect, William, *Cases of Insanity, The Epilepsy, Hypochondriacal Affection, Hysteric Passion, and Nervous Disorders, Successfully Treated* (Rochester: Fisher, 1785).

Select Cases in the Different Species of Insanity, Lunacy, or Madness, with the Modes of Practice as Adopted in the Treatment of Each (Rochester: Gillman, 1787).

Petrarch, *Petrarch's Lyric Poems*, trans. Robert M. Durling (Cambridge, MA: Harvard University Press, 1976).

Secretum, trans. J. G. Nichols (Richmond: Oneworld Classics, 2010).

Pierer, Heinrich August, *Universal-Lexikon der Vergangenheit und Gegenwart, oder Neuestes encyclopädisches Wörterbuch der Wissenschaften, Künste und Gewerbe*, 4th edn, 19 vols. (Altenburg: Pierer, 1857–65).

Pigeaud, Jackie, *Melancholia: Le malaise de l'individu* (Paris: Payot & Rivages, 2008).

'Prolégomènes à une histoire de la mélancolie', *Histoire, économie et société* 3 (1984), 501–10.

Plater, Felix, *Observationum, in hominis affectibus plerisq[ue], corpori et animo, functionum laesione, dolore, aliave molestia et vitio incommodantibus, libri tres* (Basel: Waldkirch, 1614).

Platner, Ernst, *Philosophische Aphorismen, nebst einigen Anleitungen zur philosophischen Geschichte*, 2 vols. (Leipzig: Schwickert, 1776–82).

Plutarch, *Lives I*, trans. by Bernadotte Perrin, Loeb Classical Library (London: Heinemann, 1914).

Pormann, Peter E., and Emilie Savage-Smith, *Medieval Islamic Medicine* (Edinburgh University Press, 2007).

Porter, Roy, *The Greatest Benefit to Mankind: A Medical History of Humanity from Antiquity to the Present* (London: HarperCollins, 1997).

A Social History of Madness: Stories of the Insane (New York: Weidenfeld, 1987).

Pushkin, Alexander, *Eugene Onegin*, trans. Charles Johnson (Harmondsworth: Penguin, 1979).

Pylyshyn, Z. W., *Computation and Cognition* (Cambridge, MA: MIT Press, 1984).

Pyszczynski, Tom, and Jeff Greenberg, 'Evidence for a Depressive Self-Focusing Style', *Journal of Research in Personality* 20 (1986), 95–106.

Radden, Jennifer, 'Is This Dame Melancholy? Equating Today's Depression and Past Melancholia', *Philosophy, Psychiatry, & Psychology* 10 (2003), 37–52.

The Nature of Melancholy: From Aristotle to Kristeva (New York: Oxford University Press, 2000).

Read, Rupert, 'On Approaching Schizophrenia Through Wittgenstein', *Philosophical Psychology* 14 (2001), 449–75.

Reichenbach, Hans, 'On Probability and Induction', *Philosophy of Science* 5 (1938), 21–45.

Richards, Ruth, *et al.*, 'Creativity in Manic-Depressives, Cyclothymes, Their Normal Relatives, and Control Subjects', *Journal of Abnormal Psychology* 1988 (97), 281–8.

Richardson, Tim, *The Arcadian Friends: Inventing the English Landscape Garden* (London: Bantam, 2008).

Rosen, George, 'Nostalgia: A "Forgotten" Psychological Disorder', *Psychological Medicine* 5 (1975), 340–54.

Rousseau, Jean-Jacques, *Dictionnaire de Musique*, in *Collection complète des œuvres de J. J. Rousseau*, ed. Pierre-Alexandre du Peyrou and Paul Moultou (Geneva: Société Typographique, 1780–9).

Rubin, Julius H., *Religious Melancholy and Protestant Experience in America* (Oxford University Press, 1994).

Rufus of Ephesus, *On Melancholy*, ed. Peter E. Pormann, SAPERE XII (Tübingen: Mohr Siebeck, 2008).

Ryder, Andrew G., *et al.*, 'The Cultural Shaping of Depression: Somatic Symptoms in China, Psychological Symptoms in North America?', *Journal of Abnormal Psychology* 117 (2008), 300–13.

Sartorius, N., *et al.*, *Depressive Disorders in Different Cultures: Report on the WHO Collaborative Study on Standardized Assessment of Depressive Disorders* (Geneva: World Health Organization, 1983), 92.

Sass, Louis A., *The Paradoxes of Delusion: Wittgenstein, Schreber, and the Schizophrenic Mind* (Ithaca, NY: Cornell University Press, 1994).

Schalk, Fritz, 'Der Artikel "mélancolie" in der Diderot'schen Enzyklopädie', in Schalk, *Studien zur französischen Aufklärung* (Frankfurt/Main: Klostermann, 1977), 206–20.

Schär, Markus, *Seelennöte der Untertanen. Selbstmord, Melancholie und Religion im Alten Zürich, 1500–1800* (Zürich: Chronos, 1985).

Schiesari, Juliana, *The Gendering of Melancholia: Feminism, Psychoanalysis, and the Symbolics of Loss in Renaissance Literature* (Ithaca, NY: Cornell University Press, 1992).

Schiller, Friedrich, *The Robbers*, in Schiller, *The Robbers and Wallenstein*, trans. F. J. Lamport (Harmondsworth: Penguin, 1979).

Werke. Nationalausgabe, ed. Julius Petersen *et al.* (Stuttgart: Böhlau, 1943 ff.).

Schleiner, Winfried, *Melancholy, Genius and Utopia in the Renaissance* (Wiesbaden: Harrassowitz, 1991).

Schmidt, Jeremy, *Melancholy and the Care of the Soul: Religion, Moral Philosophy and Madness in Early Modern England* (Aldershot: Ashgate, 2007).

Schoevers, R. A., *et al.*, 'Risk Factors for Depression in Later Life: Results of a Prospective Community Based Study', *Journal of Affective Disorders* 59 (2000), 127–37.

Schöner, Erich, *Das Viererschema in der antiken Humoralpathologie*, Südhoffs Archiv Beiheft 4 (Wiesbaden: Steiner, 1964).

Scottish ECT Accreditation Network Annual Report 2009. Reporting on *2008* (Edinburgh: NHS National Services Scotland, 2009).

Screech, M. A., *Montaigne and Melancholy: The Wisdom of the Essays* (London: Duckworth, 1983).

Scull, Andrew T., *Hysteria: The Biography* (Oxford University Press, 2009).

Seligman, Martin E. P., *Learned Helplessness: On Depression, Development, and Death* (San Francisco: Freeman, 1975).

Shakespeare, William, *Complete Works*, ed. Richard Proudfoot, Ann Thompson, and David Scott Kastan, rev. edn (London: The Arden Shakespeare, 2001).

Shorter, Edward, *Before Prozac: The Troubled History of Mood Disorders in Psychiatry* (Oxford University Press, 2009).

  'The Doctrine of the Two Depressions in Historical Perspective', *Acta Psychiatrica Scandinavica* 115, suppl. 433 (2007), 5–13.

  A History of Psychiatry: From the Era of the Asylum to the Age of Prozac (New York: Wiley, 1997).

Showalter, Elaine, *The Female Malady: Women, Madness, and English Culture, 1830–1980* (London: Virago, 1987).

Sickels, Eleanor Maria, *The Gloomy Egoist: Moods and Themes of Melancholy from Gray to Keats*, Columbia University Studies in English and Comparative Literature (New York: Columbia University Press, 1932).

Skultans, Vieda, *English Madness: Ideas on Insanity, 1580–1890* (London: Routledge & Kegan Paul, 1979).

Smith, Charlotte, *Celestina*, 2nd edn (London: Cadell, 1791).

  Emmeline; Or the Orphan of the Castle (London: Cadell, 1788).

  Etheline; Or the Recluse of the Lake (London: Cadell, 1789).

  Desmond (London: Robinson, 1792).

  The Old Manor House (London: Bell, 1793).

  Marchmont (London: Low, 1796).

  Montalbert (London: Low, 1795).

  The Wanderings of Warwick (London: Bell, 1794).

Smolen, Robert C., 'Expectancies, Mood, and Performance of Depressed and Nondepressed Psychiatric Inpatients on Chance and Skill Tasks', *Journal of Abnormal Psychology* 87 (1978), 91–101.

Solomon, Andrew, *The Noonday Demon: An Anatomy of Depression* (London: Vintage, 2002).

Southey, Robert, *The Poetical Works of Robert Southey, Collected by Himself*, 10 vols. (Longman: London, 1837).

Stachniewski, John, *The Persecutory Imagination: English Puritanism and the Literature of Religious Despair* (Oxford University Press, 1991), 27.

Stern, J. P., 'The Dear Purchase', *German Quarterly* 41 (1968), 317–37.

  The Dear Purchase: A Theme in German Modernism (Cambridge University Press, 1995).

Stone, Lawrence, *The Family, Sex and Marriage in England, 1500–1800*, abridged edn (London: Penguin, 1990).

Summers, R. W., R. J. Dawson, and R. E. Phillips, 'Assortative Mating and Patterns of Inheritance Indicate That the Three Crossbill Taxa in Scotland Are Species', *Journal of Avian Biology* 38 (2007), 153–62.

Szasz, Thomas, *Law, Liberty, and Psychiatry: An Inquiry into the Social Uses of Mental Health Practices* (New York: Macmillan, 1963).

Schizophrenia: The Sacred Symbol of Psychiatry (Syracuse, NY: Syracuse University Press, 1988).

Tang, C. S., and J. W. Critelli, 'Depression and Judgment of Control: Impact of a Contingency on Accuracy', *Journal of Personality* 58 (1990), 717–27.

Tawney, R. H., 'Preface' in Max Weber, *The Protestant Ethic and the Spirit of Capitalism*, trans. Talcott Parsons (London: Allen & Unwin, 1930).

Religion and the Rise of Capitalism: A Historical Study (London: Murray, 1926).

Taylor, Charles, *Sources of the Self: The Making of Modern Identity* (Cambridge University Press, 1989).

Taylor, Michael Alan, and Max Fink, *Melancholia: The Diagnosis, Pathophysiology and Treatment of Depressive Illness* (Cambridge University Press, 2006).

Taylor, Shelley E., and Jonathon D. Brown, 'Illusion and Well-Being', *Psychological Bulletin* 103 (1988), 193–210.

Temkin, Owsei, *Galenism: Rise and Decline of a Medical Philosophy* (Ithaca, NY: Cornell University Press, 1973).

Thiher, Allen, *Revels in Madness: Insanity in Medicine and Literature* (Ann Arbor, MI: University of Michigan Press, 1999).

Thomas, Keith, *Religion and the Decline of Magic* (Harmondsworth: Penguin, 1971).

Tolkien, J. R. R., *The Lord of the Rings* (London: HarperCollins, 1995).

Tomkins, Silvan S., *Affect, Imagery and Consciousness*, 4 vols. (New York: Springer, 1962–92).

Treffert, D. A., 'The Savant Syndrome: An Extraordinary Condition. A Synopsis: Past, Present, Future', *Philosophical Transactions of the Royal Society of London. Series B: Biological Sciences* 364 (2009), 1351–7.

Tsouna, Voula, 'Epicurean therapeutic strategies', *The Cambridge Companion to Epicureanism*, ed. James Warren (Cambridge University Press, 2009), 249–65.

Tuan, Yi-fu, *Segmented Worlds and Self: Group Life and Individual Consciousness* (Minneapolis, MN: University of Minnesota Press, 1982).

Tversky, Amos, and Daniel Kahneman, 'Judgment Under Uncertainty: Heuristics and Biases', *Science* 185/4157 (1974), 1124–31.

Ugarte, Eduardo, 'The Demoniacal Impulse: The Construction of Amok in the Philippines', unpublished dissertation, University of Western Sydney, 1999.

Ullmann, Manfred, *Islamic Medicine* (Edinburgh University Press, 1978).

Valk, Thorsten, *Melancholie im Werk Goethes* (Tübingen: Niemeyer, 2002).

Vogel, Claus, 'Zur Entstehung der hippokratischen Viersäftelehre', unpublished dissertation, University of Marburg, 1956.

Walker Bynum, Caroline, 'Did the Twelfth Century Discover the Individual?', *Journal of Ecclesiastical History* 31 (1980), 1–17.

Waugh, Linda, 'Marked and Unmarked: A Choice Between Unequals in Semiotic Structure', *Semiotica* 38 (1982), 299–318.

Weber, Max, *The Protestant Ethic and the Spirit of Capitalism*, trans. Talcott Parsons, with an introduction by Anthony Giddens (London: Routledge, 1992).

Weissman, Myrna, *et al.*, 'Cross-National Epidemiology of Major Depression and Bipolar Disorder', *Journal of the American Medical Association* 276 (1996), 293–9.

Wenzel, Siegfried, *The Sin of Sloth: Acedia in Medieval Thought and Literature* (Chapel Hill, NC: University of North Carolina Press, 1967).

Wilson, S. H., and G. M. Walker, 'Unemployment and Health: A Review', *Public Health* 107 (1993), 153–62.

Winzeler, Robert L., *Latah in South-East Asia: The History and Ethnography of a Culture-Bound Syndrome* (Cambridge University Press, 1995).

Wolpert, Lewis, *Malignant Sadness: The Anatomy of Depression* (London: Faber and Faber, 1999).

Wurtzel, Elizabeth, *Prozac Nation: Young and Depressed in America*, 2nd edn (London: Quartet Books, 1996).

Zachar, Peter, 'Psychiatric Disorders Are Not Natural Kinds', *Philosophy, Psychiatry, & Psychology* 7 (2000), 167–82.

Zedler, Johann Heinrich, *Grosses vollständiges Universal-Lexicon aller Wissenschafften und Künste, welche bishero durch menschlichen Verstand und Witz erfunden und verbessert worden*, 66 vols. (Leipzig and Halle: Zedler, 1732–52).

Index

Abramson, Lyn, 157–60
acedia, 110
Adair, James Makittrick, 74
Aëtius of Amida, 45, 64, 178
Alexander of Tralles, 45
Alloy, Lauren, 156–60
amok, 102
Anaximander, 24
Anaximenes, 24
Arctinus of Miletus, 49
Aretaeus of Cappadocia, 42, 64, 67, 79
Aristophanes, 39
Aristotle, 11, 27, 39, 42, 48, 80–1, 85, 88, 94, 95, 96, 132, 134, 152, 179
asthenia, 52, 75, 114
ataques de nervios, 102
autism, 30, 78
Avicenna (Ibn Sīnā), 46

Barnard, Sir John, 144
Baxter, Richard, 122
Beck, Aaron T., 158
Beethoven, Ludwig van, 162
Bellerophontes, 110
Benjamin, Walter, 170
Berkeley, George, 107
Bible, the, 23, 84, 92, 110, 162, 179, 180
Blair, Hugh, 172
Bloor, David, 5
Boccherini, Luigi, 162
Boerhaave, Herman, 73
Borch-Jacobsen, Mikkel, 4, 18
Boyd, Richard, 16, 17, 20
Bright, Timothie, 138
Burckhardt, Jacob, 118, 125, 126, 129
Burns, Robert, 124
Burton, Robert, 53, 60, 64, 79, 87, 88, 93, 95, 104, 105, 109, 110, 138, 140, 141, 172, 178
Byron, George Gordon, Lord, 153, 175, 187

Calvin, Jean, 119
capitalism, 31
Carothers, J. C., 101
Carpzov, Benedikt, 88
Caston, Victor, 132
Caxton, William, 139
Celsus, 42
Chabrier, Emmanuel, 162
Chartier, Alain, 83
Cheyne, George, 94, 105–7, 108, 122, 146, 168
Cicero, 166
comorbidity, 12–13
Constantinus Africanus, 32, 45, 46, 139
constructivism
    psychiatric, 7, 8, 15
    social, 8–9
Cooper, Rachel, 20
Cranach the Elder, Lukas, 83
Crato von Krafftheim, Johannes, 60
Cullen, William, 61, 74

Dante Alighieri, 130
Darwin, Charles, 16
Davies, John, 132
Dawkins, Richard, 16
Democritus, 27
depression
    creativity and, 153–6
    cultural difference and, 98–9, 100–4
    etymology of, 48–51
    gender and, 76–8
    melancholic, 56
    of spirits, 51–2
    socio-economics of, 115–18
    therapies for, 56–8
depressive realism, 156–60
Descartes, René, 28, 167
Diderot, Denis, 170
Dienstag, Joshua Foa, 30, 137
Diocles of Carystus, 133